Inclusive Mental Health Practice

A Practical Guide for Nurses and Therapists Working with Culturally Diverse Patients

I0027079

Theo Seki

The information presented in "Inclusive Mental Health Practice: A Practical Guide for Nurses and Therapists working with culturally diverse Patients" is intended for educational and informational purposes only. It is designed to offer general guidance and best practices for healthcare professionals working in mental health.

This book is not a substitute for professional medical, psychological, or therapeutic advice, diagnosis, or treatment. Readers are urged to consult with qualified healthcare professionals for any specific health concerns, diagnoses, or treatment plans. The application of the principles discussed in this book should always be adapted to individual patient needs, clinical judgment, and current professional guidelines and ethical standards.

While every effort has been made to ensure the accuracy and completeness of the information within this publication, the healthcare field is constantly evolving. Therefore, the author and publisher disclaim any liability for any errors, omissions, or consequences arising from the use of the information contained herein.

Any individuals, organizations, or case scenarios mentioned or alluded to within this book are entirely fictitious and are used for illustrative purposes only. They do not represent any real persons, living or deceased, or actual organizations or events. Any resemblance to real individuals or entities is purely coincidental. The use of hypothetical situations is intended to facilitate learning and discussion without infringing upon the privacy or identity of any real persons or groups.

The author and publisher are not responsible for the misuse or misinterpretation of the content within this book. Readers are encouraged to apply the knowledge gained responsibly and ethically within their professional scope of practice.

ISBN: 978-1-7641942-4-2
Isohan Publishing

Table of Contents

Chapter 1: The Call for Cultural Care in Mental Health

Defining Cultural Ways: Competence, Humility, and Sensitivity

Providing helpful mental health care in a connected world starts with knowing some key ideas. **Cultural competence** often means learning specific facts, skills, and ways of thinking that help a clinician care for people from all sorts of backgrounds. That's a good start, but it's really just the beginning of a longer journey.

A better way to think about it is **cultural humility**. This isn't a destination you arrive at, but a promise you make to yourself for life: to always check your own thoughts and habits, to admit what you don't know, and to really try to see things from your patient's viewpoint. It means working *with* your patient, not just *for* them, creating a partnership where you both share in making choices. This change from just "being competent" to "practicing humility" changes everything. It's about more than just gathering facts; it's about evening out power differences and building trusting, non-judgmental relationships. This isn't just a nice idea; it's a moral must-do for fair and equal care. **Cultural sensitivity**, a close cousin, is simply being aware of and respecting differences in culture. It's the groundwork for both competence and humility.

The World's Changing Face and Mental Health Practice

Today's societies are changing fast. More and more people are moving between countries, and our own communities are becoming more varied within their borders. This change means mental health professionals absolutely must learn to offer care that respects culture. The truth is, a person's culture and background greatly shape how they experience mental health struggles, how they show distress, and how they connect with treatment. If societies keep getting more diverse, then old ways of doing mental health care—

ways that often only considered one main culture—just won't work as well. The types of concerns patients bring and how they react to therapy are different now, and that makes truly skilled, culturally informed care a fundamental requirement. This shows that the need for cultural understanding isn't a passing fad; it's a deep, growing necessity driven by how our world is changing.

Case Example 1: Mr. Lee and the "Heart Problem"

Mr. Lee, a 68-year-old immigrant from rural Vietnam, was sent to a community mental health clinic by his general doctor. He complained of severe chest pain, shortness of breath, and feeling tired all the time. His general doctor had run many tests, but found no physical reason for his symptoms. The therapist, a young woman new to the area, saw in Mr. Lee's chart that he was diagnosed with generalized anxiety disorder by the referring doctor. During their first meeting, Mr. Lee barely made eye contact and spoke softly, mostly about his physical problems. He kept saying, "My heart feels bad, like a heavy stone." He never used words like "anxiety" or "worry." The therapist, worried about missing something, asked, "Mr. Lee, when you say your heart feels bad, what else is happening? Are you feeling nervous or scared?" Mr. Lee just shook his head.

Later, the therapist discussed the case with a more experienced colleague. The colleague explained that in many East Asian cultures, emotional distress, especially anxiety or sadness, often shows up as physical symptoms – this is called **somatization**. Directly asking about "anxiety" might not make sense to someone who experiences their distress in their body. She suggested asking about "nervousness in the stomach" or "trouble sleeping because of too many thoughts."

The next session, the therapist tried a new approach. Instead of focusing on "feelings," she asked, "Mr. Lee, what makes your body feel heavy? What worries do you carry in your mind that make your chest hurt?" Slowly, Mr. Lee started talking about his grown children, who were struggling financially, and his guilt about not being able to help them more. He worried about bringing shame to his family. This conversation, started from a place of cultural understanding of

2

somatization, opened the door to his true worries. The therapist shifted from trying to get him to name an emotion to helping him connect his physical symptoms to his life pressures, a more culturally acceptable way for him to talk about his suffering.

Understanding Differences and Fairness in Mental Health

Even with many advances in mental health care, big differences remain in who can get help, the quality of that help, and how well people from different racial and ethnic backgrounds do. These differences are not by chance. They come from a mix of problems with the system, individual biases, and cultural reasons that keep people from getting care. System problems can include unfair treatment within healthcare and not enough providers who understand different cultures. Seeing these widespread differences, and knowing how important cultural humility is, directly shapes why this book is so needed.

The problem of unfairness isn't just about what one clinician does; it's deeply part of bigger societal structures and individual professional leanings. Because the issue has many sides, fixing it needs many different actions. That's why building cultural understanding, as this guide shows, isn't just about helping one patient better. It's a key part of a bigger, urgent push to fix unfairness in the system and bring justice to public health. This means you, through your daily practice, are helping a larger movement for fair healthcare.

Case Example 2: Maria and the Language Barrier

Maria, a 30-year-old single mother from El Salvador, sought help for severe depression after losing her job. She spoke very little English, and the intake coordinator at the community clinic, short on Spanish-speaking staff, used a family member, Maria's 12-year-old daughter, to translate during the initial assessment. The daughter, eager to help her mother, often simplified Maria's complex feelings and even added her own interpretations. For example, when Maria described feeling "muerta por dentro" (dead inside), her daughter translated it as "Mom feels sad." The therapist, relying on this translation, prescribed an antidepressant and scheduled follow-up appointments.

However, Maria often missed appointments, and her symptoms did not get better. The therapist felt frustrated, wondering if Maria was not "motivated" to get better. During a team meeting, a social worker suggested using a professional, certified medical interpreter. During the next session, with the interpreter present, Maria was able to describe her intense feelings of hopelessness, profound grief over leaving her family behind, and a deep sense of shame about her unemployment. She explained that in her culture, mental illness was often seen as a weakness or a spiritual punishment, and she felt ashamed for her daughter to hear her deepest struggles. She had hesitated to speak openly with her daughter translating.

With a proper interpreter, the therapist could hear the depth of Maria's distress and her cultural beliefs about mental illness. The therapist then adjusted the treatment plan to include family counseling, where the stigma could be addressed, and connected Maria to community resources that provided support groups for Latina mothers. This experience highlighted how crucial professional interpretation is for both clear communication and building trust, especially when sensitive cultural norms are at play.

Good Practices and Your Responsibilities in Diverse Settings

Beyond just making treatment work, there's a clear ethical obligation for mental health professionals to offer care that respects culture. Professional rules for conduct always talk about doing good, doing no harm, and being fair — all of which are directly affected by how well a clinician handles cultural differences. Giving care that is respectful, works well, and is fair to all sorts of people is a basic responsibility for your profession.

Case Example 3: Ahmed and Family Involvement

Ahmed, a 22-year-old engineering student from a conservative Middle Eastern family, was referred for therapy after experiencing panic attacks during exams. He was quiet in sessions and seemed reluctant to talk about his personal life or family dynamics, often saying, "My family wouldn't understand." The therapist, trained in a Western individualistic approach, focused on helping Ahmed build independence and express his own feelings.

After several weeks with little progress, Ahmed's father called the clinic, expressing concern and asking to speak with the therapist. The therapist, mindful of patient confidentiality and Ahmed's apparent desire for privacy, politely declined to discuss the specifics of Ahmed's treatment but offered to explain the general process of therapy. The father became upset, stating, "In our culture, the family is very involved. We make decisions together. How can you help my son if you don't talk to us?"

The therapist then consulted with a supervisor who had experience with Middle Eastern cultures. The supervisor explained that for many, family collective identity is stronger than individual identity, and health decisions often involve the whole family. They suggested offering a family session, with Ahmed's permission, to discuss general goals and the role of therapy, without forcing Ahmed to share anything he wasn't comfortable with.

With Ahmed's agreement, a family session was held. The therapist explained the purpose of therapy in broad terms, emphasizing how it could help Ahmed manage stress and succeed in his studies, which resonated with the family's values. The father, feeling included and respected, then shared his own anxieties about Ahmed's future. This opened a new door. Ahmed, seeing his father's willingness to share, felt more comfortable talking about the immense academic pressure he felt from his family and his fear of disappointing them. The family session became a way to bridge cultural expectations about individualism versus collectivism, ultimately strengthening Ahmed's engagement in therapy and allowing for a more culturally fitting approach to his anxiety.

Chapter 1: Important Points

- **Cultural understanding is a must**: Modern society needs mental health care that recognizes and respects different cultures.

- **Beyond just "knowing"**: **Cultural humility** is a lifelong promise to self-check and learn from your patients, moving past just collecting facts about cultures.

- **Societal shifts require new skills**: As the world becomes more varied, traditional approaches to mental health care are not enough; new skills are needed.

- **Fairness matters**: Big differences in mental health care for different groups are real and show the need for care that addresses these problems.

- **It's your duty**: Providing culturally respectful and effective care is a core ethical and professional responsibility for all mental health workers.

Chapter 2: Culture, Identity, and Your Mental Well-being

Understanding yourself—and others—means looking at all the things that make up who we are. It means really getting how deeply these parts of us shape our mental health, how we experience illness, and how we find our way back to health. This chapter aims to untangle some of that.

Discovering Culture's Many Sides: Ethnicity, Race, Religion, Social Standing, Gender Identity, Sexual Orientation, Disability, and More

The word "culture" stretches out far beyond just where someone comes from or their nationality. It includes many different social identifiers that all together shape how a person sees the world, what they experience, and who they feel they are. These parts include **race, religion, social standing, gender identity, sexual orientation, disability status, where they grew up, and much more**. Seeing these many different parts is crucial because people often have many cultural identities at the same time. This idea, called **intersectionality**, shows how these different parts mix to create unique experiences of good fortune or hardship, deeply affecting a person's mental health and how they interact with health care systems. Acknowledging this richness is fundamental to giving truly personal and culturally fitting care.

The Place of Spirituality and Old Ways of Thinking in Health and Healing

Spirituality and long-held ways of thinking often play a big, though often missed, part in how a person approaches health and sickness. This guide directly talks about how spirituality connects with mental health. For many cultures, these beliefs shape how they see the causes of sickness, what they do to cope, and the healing methods they prefer. If you ignore or dismiss these deeply held beliefs, it can lead to a lack of trust, not following treatment plans, and in the end, worse results.

On the flip side, respectfully bringing these beliefs into treatment plans, when it's right to do so, can greatly help a patient connect with care and make the healing relationship stronger. This shows a direct connection: knowing and using a patient's spiritual or old ways of thinking not only builds trust and teamwork but also makes the treatment work better overall. This means cultural understanding isn't just about not upsetting someone; it's about actively using a patient's view of the world as a possible help for healing and connection. So, seeing the whole patient means including their spiritual and traditional beliefs, knowing they can be key parts of feeling well and getting better.

Case Example 1: Mrs. Chang's Spiritual Journey

Mrs. Chang, a 75-year-old Chinese American woman, was referred for depression after her husband passed away. She complained of feeling "empty," having trouble sleeping, and a loss of interest in her usual activities. During the initial session, she talked about her deep sadness but also mentioned visiting a Buddhist temple frequently and consulting with a traditional healer recommended by her family. The therapist, while acknowledging Mrs. Chang's grief, focused primarily on cognitive behavioral techniques to challenge negative thoughts.

After a few weeks, Mrs. Chang's depression had not lessened. She seemed polite but distant. The therapist, feeling a disconnect, asked, "Mrs. Chang, you mentioned going to the temple and seeing a healer. How do these practices help you cope with your feelings?" Mrs. Chang's face brightened. She explained that her Buddhist practice taught her about the cycle of life and death, helping her to accept loss. The traditional healer had given her herbal teas and performed rituals to cleanse her spirit, which she felt brought her peace. She explained, "These are how my people heal. They calm my spirit."

The therapist then adjusted her approach. Instead of just focusing on thoughts, she discussed how Mrs. Chang's spiritual practices could be integrated into her coping strategies. They talked about mindfulness from a Buddhist perspective, connecting it to practices of meditation she already knew. The therapist also asked if Mrs. Chang found it helpful to talk about her visits to the temple or her traditional healer, seeing them as part of her healing journey rather than separate from it. By respecting and including Mrs. Chang's spiritual framework, the therapist built a much stronger bond, and Mrs. Chang felt truly seen. This allowed her to open up more freely about her grief, leading to much better progress.

Moving to a New Culture and its Mental Health Effects

Acculturation is how people change culturally and psychologically when different cultures meet. **Assimilation** is when a person or group starts to look and act like another group in language or culture. These processes, especially for people who move to a new country or are refugees, often bring many mental health hurdles. These can include hard times before moving, the stress of getting used to a new culture (called **acculturative stress**), facing unfair treatment, and the plain difficulties of figuring out new social rules and health care systems.

This mix of things shows that the mental health of these groups is affected by a complicated blend of past events, ongoing stress from adapting, unfair societal views, and problems with the system. It shows that mental health problems are rarely just one thing, but often a complex picture of past and present difficulties, going beyond just what's in a person's head to include the bigger social and system environments. Because of this, you need to understand the many sides of what stresses a patient. You need to move beyond just giving a diagnosis to forming a full picture of the person, including their body, mind, social life, and culture, that knows about these bigger system effects. This broader understanding can also help you think about how you might help in bigger ways, like speaking up for groups of people.

Case Example 2: The Al-Hassan Family's New Home

The Al-Hassan family, refugees from Syria, arrived in the United States after years in a refugee camp. The parents, Mr. and Mrs. Al-Hassan, struggled with symptoms of depression and PTSD, but their eldest son, 17-year-old Omar, seemed to be thriving in school. The local mental health clinic was offering group therapy for refugee families, focusing on processing trauma and learning coping skills. Omar attended readily, participating actively, but his parents were hesitant. They often missed sessions, citing transportation issues or feeling "too tired."

A culturally informed outreach worker from the clinic visited the family's home. She learned that Mr. Al-Hassan felt a deep sense of loss of his traditional role as provider and protector; he was unemployed and struggling to learn English. Mrs. Al-Hassan, though appreciative of the safety, felt isolated and missed her extended family, who were still overseas. Critically, she mentioned that in Syria, mental health problems were often seen as a weakness or a sign of poor religious faith, and discussing family issues with strangers was highly frowned upon. Omar, on the other hand, was rapidly **assimilating**; he was learning English quickly, making friends at school, and embracing some American customs, which sometimes caused friction at home. His parents worried he was losing his "Syrian ways."

The outreach worker realized the group therapy model wasn't fitting their cultural needs or their **acculturative stress**. She suggested individual sessions for the parents first, where they could talk about their losses and adjust to their new roles without feeling exposed. She also helped them connect with a local Syrian community center, which offered language classes and cultural events, helping them feel less isolated. For Omar, she helped the family find a school-based program that could talk about **acculturation** challenges and cultural identity, helping both Omar and his parents understand his changing identity. This approach, which met the family where they were culturally and addressed the specific stresses of adjusting to a new way of life, slowly built trust and allowed the family to begin their healing process more effectively.

Knowing About Shame and How People Seek Help Across Cultures

What a culture believes about mental sickness deeply changes how much shame is tied to it, which then affects whether people will seek help. In some cultures, mental health problems might be seen as a fault in character, a curse from spirits, or something that brings shame to the family. This can make people put off getting professional help or rely on healers from their own traditions. Beyond that, how people show psychological distress is very different from one culture to another. What might be called anxiety or sadness in a Western setting could show up as body pains (called **somatization**) or other culturally specific ways of showing distress in another. Knowing these differences is critical for accurately seeing, diagnosing, and helping in the right way.

Case Example 3: The Patel Family and "Nerves"

Mrs. Patel, a 45-year-old woman from India living with her extended family in a Midwestern city, was brought to a clinic by her eldest son. He explained that his mother had been suffering from "nerves" for months. Mrs. Patel herself described constant headaches, stomach upset, and a feeling of "heat" in her head. She reported trouble sleeping and said she felt "heavy" all the time. She denied feeling sad or anxious, stating firmly, "I don't have sadness; I have nerves." The physician, seeing no physical cause for her symptoms, suggested psychological counseling.

During her first session with the therapist, Mrs. Patel seemed hesitant. She avoided eye contact when the therapist asked about her emotions, and insisted her problems were "physical." The therapist learned that in Mrs. Patel's community, discussions of mental illness were rare and often carried a strong stigma. Expressing emotional distress openly could be seen as a sign of weakness or even as disrespecting the family's honor. Instead, physical complaints were a more acceptable way to voice suffering. The phrase "nerves" (or *ghabrahat* in Hindi) was a common way to talk about various forms of emotional distress without naming a mental illness.

The therapist adjusted her approach. Instead of pushing Mrs. Patel to talk about "feelings" directly, she affirmed Mrs. Patel's experience of "nerves" and focused on how these "physical symptoms" were affecting her daily life. They discussed stress reduction techniques, focusing on relaxation and improving sleep, which Mrs. Patel found acceptable because it related to her body. Slowly, as trust built, and as the therapist respected her cultural way of describing distress, Mrs. Patel began to share more. She eventually admitted that the "nerves" had worsened after a conflict with her sister-in-law, which was causing her great emotional strain and worry. By understanding the cultural expressions of distress and the stigma surrounding mental illness in her community, the therapist could meet Mrs. Patel where she was, allowing her to eventually address the deeper emotional issues in a way that felt safe and respectful to her.

Chapter 2: Important Points

- **Culture is wide-ranging**: Culture goes beyond just where someone is from; it includes race, religion, social standing, gender, sexuality, and more.

- **Spirituality matters**: A person's spiritual or old beliefs are a big part of their health journey and should be respectfully included in care.

- **New cultures bring new stresses**: Moving to a new culture creates unique mental health problems, like stress from adapting and facing unfair treatment.

- **Shame shapes seeking help**: What a culture believes about mental sickness strongly affects how much shame is felt and how—or if—people will seek professional help.

- **How distress is shown varies**: Be aware that people show mental pain differently across cultures, often through physical symptoms or special phrases.

A Final Notion for Your Path

As you hold this guide, remember that true understanding is a journey, not a destination. Each person you meet holds a universe of experiences, shaped by their culture, their history, and their spirit. Your willingness to listen, to learn, and to adapt is your greatest tool. It is in that humble act of connection that the most profound healing begins.

Chapter 3: Culturally Informed Assessment and Diagnosis

Ready to sharpen your senses? When you meet someone for the first time in a clinical setting, you're not just looking for symptoms on a checklist. You're trying to understand a whole story, one that's colored by a person's life, their family, their beliefs, and their way of seeing the world. This is where the true detective work begins—not just diagnosing, but comprehending. This chapter will give you the magnifying glass, helping you spot those subtle, yet powerful, cultural clues that make all the difference in truly connecting with someone's experience of distress.

Beyond Our Manuals: Understanding Cultural Views of Distress

While guides like the DSM-5 give us a common language for mental health, they are only a starting point. To truly help someone, you also need to grasp the cultural setting of their problems. The DSM-5 does offer a **"Cultural Formulation Interview" (CFI)**, a tool meant to help you gather facts about the cultural context of a patient's illness. But using it well means you need a deeper hold on how cultures work.

Cultural formulations go past simply checking off symptoms. They help you understand how your patient makes sense of their illness— what they believe caused it, how they think it will progress, and what they believe will make it better. This full view is crucial for really understanding a diagnosis and giving care that truly fits the patient. If you only look at symptom lists, you might misdiagnose or completely miss what your patient is actually going through. So, understanding culture is a must for a full assessment, letting you grasp the personal and cultural meaning of distress.

Spotting Syndromes and Ways of Showing Pain Tied to Culture

Culture plays a huge part in how mental health problems are understood and shown. You need to know about **culturally-bound** syndromes—special ways of showing distress found only in certain cultures—and different ways people express problems that might not fit neatly into Western labels. For example, **susto**, a folk illness from Latin America, is seen as "fright" or "soul loss" after a scary event. Symptoms might include nervousness, trouble sleeping, sadness, wanting to be alone, and physical complaints. Then there's **ataque de nervios**, also from Latin American and Caribbean cultures, which is a reaction to high stress that can involve crying, shaking, screaming, feeling detached from reality, and even thoughts of hurting oneself. Or consider **koro**, a fear that one's private parts are shrinking into the body, found in certain Asian cultures. These are some examples of such unique problems.

A common way people show psychological problems is through **somatization**. This is when anxiety or sadness shows up mostly as physical symptoms, like headaches or stomach aches, instead of clear emotional complaints. This directly challenges the Western medical idea that physical and mental illnesses are totally separate. If you don't know about somatization or culturally-bound syndromes, you might misread symptoms, leading to the wrong diagnosis or treatment that doesn't help. Seeing these different ways of showing distress means you need to look hard at your own cultural viewpoint and be open to how illness can appear outside of common Western ideas.

For example, a person from West Africa might describe **Brain Fag Syndrome**, which mainly affects students. They might complain of difficulty focusing, memory problems, pressure or pain in their head, and eye pain. These are often linked to stress from school or spiritual reasons. For someone from Southeast Asia, you might hear about **Amok**, a sudden period of quietness followed by a burst of violent, aggressive, or deadly actions towards people and things. And in many cultures, including some parts of Asia and the Middle East, people might talk about general distress through physical complaints, rather than saying, "I feel anxious" or "I'm sad." In some groups, you might even hear about **spirit possession**, where a person's behavior or sickness is thought to be caused by an outside spirit.

Case Example 1: The Case of "Susto" and Elena

Elena, a 40-year-old Salvadoran woman, came to the clinic complaining of feeling constantly tired, having nightmares, and a deep sense of dread. She had lost weight, struggled to sleep, and felt a strange feeling of "being outside of herself." She told the therapist, "I think I have *susto*." Her previous doctor had prescribed medication for anxiety and depression, but Elena felt it wasn't helping.

The therapist, familiar with the concept of culturally-bound syndromes, asked Elena what *susto* meant to her. Elena explained that she believed her soul had left her body after a sudden, frightening car accident she witnessed a few months ago—a common belief associated with *susto* in her culture. She said, "My soul is lost, and that's why I feel this emptiness." The therapist recognized that simply treating anxiety without addressing Elena's belief about *susto* would miss the core of her distress.

The therapist worked with Elena to acknowledge her belief system. They discussed the car accident in detail, validating her experience of fright. The therapist suggested coping skills for anxiety, like breathing exercises, but framed them as ways to "invite her spirit back" or "calm her nervous system" in a way that resonated with Elena's beliefs. With Elena's permission, the therapist also helped her connect with a local curandera (traditional healer) from her community. The curandera performed a ritual to "call back" Elena's spirit, which gave Elena a sense of closure and hope. While continuing therapy to address trauma symptoms, the combination of Western approaches and culturally accepted healing practices helped Elena feel understood and respected, leading to a much better outcome than medication alone.

How to Conduct Interviews and Gather History with Cultural Awareness

Good assessment really depends on your ability to do interviews that are sensitive to culture and collect a full history. This means having skills like:

- **Building trust**: Start with greetings and gestures that fit the patient's culture. Sometimes a handshake is fine; other times, a nod or slight bow is better. Observe and mirror, but always with genuine respect.

- **Asking open-ended questions**: Ask questions that invite the patient to tell their story in their own words, bringing in their cultural background without you making guesses. Instead of "Are you feeling depressed?" try "How have things been for you lately? What kind of problems have you been experiencing?"

- **Learning about their identity**: Ask about their cultural identity, their beliefs, and their practices. For instance, "What traditions are important to you and your family?" or "Do you have any spiritual practices that help you through tough times?"

- **Knowing about family and community**: Understand how family and community play a part in the patient's life. Who makes decisions? Who provides support? In many cultures, family elders or community leaders hold great influence. Getting their permission to talk with family members, when right for the patient, can give you very useful information and help with treatment.

Case Example 2: David and Family Expectations

David, a 20-year-old student from an East African immigrant family, was having trouble sleeping and focusing on his studies. He seemed withdrawn and sad. When the therapist asked about his social life, David said he spent most of his time studying or at home. He mentioned feeling "a lot of pressure" but didn't say much more. The therapist felt David was holding back.

17

During their third session, the therapist asked David about his family's hopes for him. David then explained that his parents, who had sacrificed a lot to come to the US, expected him to become a doctor—a highly respected profession in their culture. He, however, wanted to study art, but feared disappointing his family and bringing shame to them. He was secretly taking art classes, which created a huge conflict inside him, causing his distress.

The therapist then asked, "David, in your family, who usually helps with big decisions like this?" David explained that his grandfather, still in Africa, was the most respected elder, and his father in the US also held a lot of sway. The therapist, with David's agreement, suggested that they could talk about ways to approach his family respectfully, perhaps even involving them in a broader conversation about his future (without forcing David to reveal his art passion immediately, but rather explore shared values like success and happiness). By asking about family roles and decision-making, the therapist got to the heart of David's conflict, showing how understanding family norms is key to helping a patient.

Handling Diagnostic Problems in Different Cultural Settings

Using Western diagnostic rules on people from different backgrounds can cause many problems. It can lead to too many diagnoses or not enough. You need to know how cultural norms might change how symptoms appear, which could lead to wrong interpretations. Getting extra information from family or community members, and looking at it through a cultural lens, cannot be stressed enough. In hard cases, asking for cultural advice from experts who really understand certain cultures can be very helpful for getting the right diagnosis and adjusting treatment plans.

For example, a study showed that African Americans are significantly more likely to be diagnosed with schizophrenia compared to White Americans, even when presenting with similar symptoms. One reason for this disparity, according to research, is that clinicians may misinterpret culturally typical behaviors or expressions of spiritual beliefs as psychotic symptoms [14]. Similarly, some research indicates that Latinx individuals, particularly immigrants, may be overdiagnosed with psychotic disorders and underdiagnosed with mood or anxiety disorders, due to clinicians' lack of understanding of culturally specific idioms of distress or somatization [15]. These statistics highlight how critical it is for you to be aware of your own biases and the cultural filters you apply during assessment.

Case Example 3: The Case of Mr. Chen and "Ghost Sickness"

Mr. Chen, a 55-year-old man from rural China, was brought to the emergency room by his worried adult children. He was talking to himself, seeing things that weren't there, and refused to eat, saying that "ghosts are trying to take my spirit." The emergency psychiatrist, seeing clear signs of psychosis, diagnosed him with acute schizophrenia and began standard antipsychotic medication.

After a week, Mr. Chen was still very disturbed. His children, though respectful of the doctors, quietly suggested, "Perhaps he has 'ghost sickness.' Our village elder knows how to deal with this." The hospital staff, though well-meaning, dismissed this as a superstitious belief.

A social worker with a background in cultural studies happened to be on the unit. She spoke with the family and learned that in Mr. Chen's village, sudden changes in behavior and talking to unseen entities were often explained as "ghost sickness" or a spirit imbalance. While acknowledging the Western diagnosis of psychosis, the social worker suggested a cultural consultation. A local Chinese community leader, who was also a respected elder, came to speak with Mr. Chen and his family. The elder explained the Western medical view in a culturally understandable way—that the medication was "strengthening his mind" against the "ghosts"—and performed a small, calming ritual that made Mr. Chen feel less afraid.

The combination of medication and cultural understanding made a huge difference. Mr. Chen felt his beliefs were respected, which reduced his resistance. The family felt heard and more willing to support his treatment. This case shows how important it is to not only recognize cultural explanations for illness but to find ways to bridge those explanations with Western medical treatment, sometimes by seeking outside help.

Chapter 3: Important Points

- **Beyond symptoms**: Don't just check off symptoms; understand the patient's cultural ideas about their illness.

- **Know cultural syndromes**: Learn about specific problems and ways of showing distress tied to different cultures.

- **Interview with care**: Use culturally right greetings, ask open-ended questions, and learn about family roles.

- **Watch for diagnostic traps**: Be aware that Western diagnoses might not always fit other cultures, and use cultural advice when needed.

- **Numbers show the need**: Disparities in diagnosis for certain racial and ethnic groups show how important cultural awareness is.

Chapter 4: Clear Talk and Working with Interpreters

Have you ever tried to build a house with just half the tools? That's what providing mental health care without truly clear communication feels like. It's not just about words; it's about unspoken cues, respectful silences, and knowing when a gesture means one thing here and something entirely different there. And when language itself is a barrier, well, that's when a skilled interpreter becomes your invaluable partner in bridge-building. This chapter gives you the blueprint for that bridge.

Speaking and Not Speaking: How Cultures Affect Communication

Talking is a mix of what we say and what our bodies tell. Both are deeply shaped by culture. Differences in how people talk—like being direct versus indirect, how much silence they use, how close they stand, how much eye contact they make, and their hand movements—can lead to big misunderstandings if you don't notice them. For example, looking someone directly in the eye might show honesty in one culture, but disrespect in another. You need to be aware of these small points to build trust and really understand what your patient is communicating. When non-verbal cues seem off from what's being said, always ask for more clarity.

Consider the example of **silence**. In some Western cultures, silence in a conversation can feel awkward or like resistance. However, in many Indigenous cultures or some Asian cultures, silence can mean respect, contemplation, or that a person is carefully considering their words. Interrupting this silence could be seen as rude or rushing the patient. Similarly, **eye contact** varies greatly. In some parts of the Middle East or Latin America, sustained direct eye contact with someone in authority might be avoided as a sign of respect, especially by younger individuals or women. In contrast, in mainstream American culture, avoiding eye contact might be misinterpreted as dishonesty or evasiveness.

The Best Ways to Use Professional Interpreters

When you can't speak the same language, using **professional medical interpreters** is not just helpful; it's a must. Relying on family members—especially children—or staff who are just bilingual but not trained, can cause big problems. You could get important medical facts wrong, break privacy rules, and run into serious ethical issues.

Using an interpreter correctly means following a clear plan:

1. **Before the session**: Have a quick chat with the interpreter. Tell them what you hope to do in the session, if any sensitive topics will come up, and if you'll use any special words. This helps them prepare.

2. **During the session**: When talking, keep your eyes on the patient, even when the interpreter is speaking. This helps you connect directly with the patient. Speak clearly, in shorter sentences, and avoid jargon.

3. **After the session**: Take a moment to talk with the interpreter. You can ask for clarity on anything that seemed unclear, discuss cultural specifics they noticed, and get their feedback.

This complete approach shows that working with an interpreter is a skill, not just about translating words. It's about handling the healing relationship within a "therapeutic triangle" to make sure you stay connected to your patient, even through someone else. This way of working is a key step to keep patients safe and act in a morally right way.

For instance, studies show that using ad hoc interpreters (like family or untrained staff) leads to significantly more errors than professional interpreters. One study found that ad hoc interpreters made 2.5 times more errors, with many of those errors having potential clinical consequences [16]. Another report highlighted that nearly 80% of healthcare organizations in the US still use ad hoc interpreters despite strong recommendations against it, particularly in mental health settings where nuances are critical [17]. These numbers underscore the real risks involved when professional interpreters aren't used.

Dealing with Language Differences and How We Talk

Beyond simply changing words from one language to another, you need to be aware of the small details of language differences. This means making complicated medical terms simpler, not using common sayings or comparisons that might not translate well, and always checking that the patient understands. It's also important to see how language barriers can make patients feel—they might feel frustrated, misunderstood, or like they have no say when they can't fully express themselves. Being patient, truly listening, and being willing to change how you talk are most important here.

Case Example 1: Mr. Kim and the Lost Idiom

Mr. Kim, a 60-year-old Korean immigrant, was seeing a therapist for what appeared to be symptoms of generalized anxiety. During one session, he described his worries by saying, "My heart feels like a pounding rice cake." The therapist, not understanding the idiom, politely nodded and continued, focusing on cognitive restructuring techniques. Mr. Kim seemed to disconnect after this, becoming less engaged.

Later, the therapist discussed the session with a Korean colleague.

The colleague explained that "pounding rice cake" (떡방아 찧듯) is a common Korean idiom describing a rapid, intense, and often fearful heartbeat, akin to a panic attack or extreme anxiety. It's a vivid, culturally specific way to express distress. The therapist realized she had missed a chance to validate Mr. Kim's unique expression of his feelings.

In the next session, the therapist started by saying, "Mr. Kim, last time you talked about your heart feeling like a 'pounding rice cake.' Can you tell me more about that feeling? What does that mean to you?" Mr. Kim's face visibly relaxed. He then shared how that sensation made him feel incredibly vulnerable, reminding him of times he felt helpless. By understanding and acknowledging his idiom, the therapist showed true respect for his cultural way of expressing distress, which strengthened their connection and made Mr. Kim feel more comfortable sharing his true experience.

Building Trust and Connection in Cross-Cultural Meetings

Making a strong healing connection is key to good mental health care, and this is especially true when working with people from different cultures. **Cultural humility**, which means admitting your own limits and biases, really trying to see things from your patient's side, and talking with respect, is the key to making this connection. This way of working creates a partnership instead of a boss-and-worker setup, which then builds trust and helps everyone make decisions together. Showing real interest, respect for how a patient sees the world, and a willingness to learn are powerful ways to build trust across different cultures.

Case Example 2: Fatima and the Power of Shared Space

Fatima, a young Muslim woman from Afghanistan, was seeing a male therapist for trauma related to her past. In their initial sessions, Fatima would often keep her head down, give short answers, and sit very stiffly, avoiding direct eye contact. The therapist, trained to encourage open communication and direct engagement, initially felt Fatima was resistant.

He later consulted with a female colleague who had experience with Afghan culture. She explained that for some Afghan women, particularly when speaking with a male outside their family, direct eye contact can be seen as inappropriate or too forward, and a modest demeanor is common. She also suggested that the physical setup of the room might be uncomfortable.

In the next session, the therapist made a subtle change. Instead of sitting directly across from Fatima, he angled his chair slightly,

24

creating a less confrontational posture. He also began the session by asking, "Fatima, I want to make sure you feel comfortable here. Is there anything about our space or how we talk that could make it easier for you to share?" Fatima hesitated, then softly suggested, "Perhaps if the door was a little more closed?" and "I feel better when I can look at the wall when I think." The therapist immediately closed the door fully and placed a small, decorative screen near her chair that allowed her to look away without appearing to avoid him directly. These small, culturally aware adjustments, prompted by a willingness to ask and adapt, helped Fatima feel safer and more respected. Over time, she gradually relaxed and began to share more openly, not because the therapist changed his core skills, but because he adapted their expression to fit her cultural comfort.

Case Example 3: The Rodriguez Family and Time

The Rodriguez family, recent immigrants from Colombia, came to the clinic for their son Mateo, who was having behavioral problems at school. The appointment was set for 10:00 AM, but the family arrived at 10:30 AM with several other relatives, including an elder aunt. The receptionist, accustomed to strict scheduling, seemed frustrated, and the clinician felt a rush to start the session.

During the session, the family often interrupted each other, speaking over one another with enthusiasm. The clinician, used to a more linear, turn-taking conversation style, found it hard to get a clear picture of Mateo's issues and felt overwhelmed by the multiple voices. She politely tried to regain control by saying, "One person at a time, please." The family seemed to quiet down, but then became less lively, and the conversation felt forced.

A supervisor observed the session through a one-way mirror and later spoke with the clinician. The supervisor explained that in many Latin American cultures, "clock time" is less strict than in Western cultures, and showing up a little late with extended family is not uncommon; it can even be a sign of respect and familial support. Also, in some collectivist cultures, an overlapping, dynamic conversation style is normal and shows engagement, not disrespect. The supervisor suggested that the clinician try to relax her expectations around time and communication style.

In the next family session, the clinician purposefully allowed for a more flexible start. When the family arrived, she warmly greeted each person, including the aunt, acknowledging their presence. During the discussion, she let the conversation flow more naturally, only gently guiding it when it strayed too far. She learned to listen for the overall message even amidst overlapping voices. By adapting her approach to time and communication norms, the clinician showed respect for the family's cultural style, which led to a much more productive and open discussion about Mateo's challenges, ultimately helping the family feel heard and understood.

Key Points

- **Communication is cultural**: Both what you say and how you say it (like eye contact or personal space) are shaped by culture.

- **Use professional interpreters**: For language differences, always use trained medical interpreters—it's crucial for safety and ethics.

- **Clear language is a must**: Simplify complex terms and avoid idioms that might not translate well.

- **Build trust with cultural humility**: Show respect, curiosity, and a desire to learn about your patient's world to build a strong connection.

- **Numbers speak volumes**: Studies prove that professional interpreters make fewer errors, showing their value in patient care.

Chapter 5: Making Interventions Fit the Culture

Imagine giving someone a beautifully wrapped gift, but it's the wrong size, the wrong color, and for the wrong occasion. It might be a good gift in itself, but it won't truly serve the person receiving it. The same goes for therapy. We have powerful, evidence-based tools, but without fitting them to the person and their culture, they might miss the mark. This chapter is all about taking those tools and making them just right, ensuring they truly help the unique individuals you serve.

How to Change Therapies for Culture

Cultural adaptation means changing an intervention in a planned way to consider a population's culture, setting, and language. The reason to do this is simple: therapies that work well where they started might not work, or might even be harmful, if they're not adjusted for different groups. This process means changing many things, from small tweaks like language and comparisons to bigger shifts in examples, how you deliver the therapy, and even the main ideas of the therapy, so they fit with the patient's cultural values and how they see the world.

For example, **Cognitive Behavioral Therapy (CBT)**, a widely used therapy, has been changed successfully for many cultural groups [18]. This has meant using examples that fit the culture, changing how people communicate, and dealing with cultural values tied to thoughts and feelings. For instance, in cultures that value the group over the individual, changing negative thoughts might be talked about in terms of how it helps the family or community, not just the person. This shows that changing therapy is a planned, many-sided process that can mean rethinking the very basics of therapy, not just small changes. This planned way of doing things makes sure that changes make the therapy better, not weaker, which is key for good practice in varied settings.

Research consistently shows that culturally adapted interventions are more effective than unadapted ones for minority groups. A meta-analysis of 76 studies found that culturally adapted mental health interventions had a moderate to large positive effect size compared to unadapted interventions, with even stronger effects for specific ethnic groups [19]. This indicates that adaptation isn't just a nicety; it genuinely improves outcomes.

Mixing Old Ways of Healing with Modern Medical Care

In many cultures, traditional healing and spiritual beliefs play a big part in how people approach health and sickness. Working with traditional healers in a respectful way and carefully including culturally fitting practices into treatment plans can greatly help patients connect with care and make the healing relationship stronger. These practices might include spiritual rituals, prayer, herbal medicines, or support networks from the community.

But, you need to include these beliefs respectfully and **"where appropriate."** This means you need a careful approach, not just saying yes to everything. You need guidance on how to figure out if these traditional practices fit with Western care and if they are safe. You also need to know how to handle possible disagreements between old ways and new, and how to do it ethically without taking over or disrespecting old practices. Good guides should include how to check if traditional practices work well with modern care, how to build good working relationships with traditional healers, and how to make sure patients are safe and can make their own choices about their care.

Case Example 1: Mr. Ibrahim and Cupping Therapy

Mr. Ibrahim, a 50-year-old immigrant from Egypt, was receiving medication and talk therapy for chronic back pain and related depression. He respectfully informed his therapist that he also regularly sought "cupping therapy" (Hijama) from a traditional practitioner in his community, believing it helped release "bad blood" and brought balance to his body and spirit. His medical doctor, unaware of this, had expressed concern about potential bruising.

The therapist, recalling the importance of integrating traditional practices when appropriate, asked Mr. Ibrahim more about cupping. Mr. Ibrahim explained it was an ancient Islamic practice that provided both physical relief and spiritual cleansing. He felt it was a vital part of his healing. The therapist then researched cupping therapy, learning that while it might cause bruising, it was generally considered safe when done by a skilled practitioner.

Instead of dismissing it, the therapist had an open conversation with Mr. Ibrahim. "Mr. Ibrahim," she said, "I understand that cupping is important to you and helps you feel better. My goal is to make sure all your treatments work well together and keep you safe." She asked him to keep her informed about his cupping sessions and to tell his traditional practitioner about his Western medical care. She also used the concept of "balance" that Mr. Ibrahim valued to frame their talk therapy sessions, discussing how addressing his emotional pain could also help him achieve spiritual and physical balance. By accepting and understanding his traditional practice, the therapist strengthened their trust, and Mr. Ibrahim felt more comfortable sharing other aspects of his health, leading to a more unified approach to his care.

Family Ways and Community Help in Treatment

The idea that the "person" is the main focus of care, common in Western psychology, might not fit with cultures where the family or community is the central group. Knowing the role of family and community in different cultures is key for planning good treatment. This means learning about cultural rules for privacy, who makes decisions in the family, and the role of older family members or community leaders. Having family members help with treatment, if the patient agrees and it's right to do so, can give very helpful support and help patients stick with their plan. But, you must do this in a way that respects the culture and honors how the family already works.

For example, in many Asian cultures, including Chinese and Vietnamese, family interdependence is a strong value. Decisions about health are often made collectively, or heavily influenced by elders, rather than solely by the individual. A study examining mental health help-seeking among Vietnamese Americans found that family cohesion and approval significantly impacted an individual's willingness to engage in therapy [20]. Ignoring this could lead to patients feeling isolated from their family or even dropping out of treatment because it conflicts with their family values.

Medicine Choices for Different Groups

Giving medicines also needs cultural thought. Beliefs about mental health drugs, including how well they work, their side effects, and the shame linked to them, are very different across cultures and can greatly affect whether someone takes their medicine as prescribed. Beyond that, genetic differences across ethnic groups can change how drugs are processed in the body, affecting how much medicine is needed and what side effects might happen. You need to know about these possible differences and talk openly with patients about their beliefs and experiences with medicine to get the best treatment results.

For example, genetic differences can impact how individuals metabolize certain psychiatric medications. About 1 in 15 White Americans, 1 in 5 African Americans, and 1 in 20 East Asians are considered "poor metabolizers" of certain common antidepressants like SSRIs due to variations in the CYP2D6 enzyme [21]. This means they might need lower doses or experience more side effects than other groups. Conversely, some groups, like people of East Asian descent, can be "ultrarapid metabolizers" of certain antipsychotics, meaning they might need higher doses for the drug to be effective [22]. These variations are not just interesting facts; they have direct consequences for how you prescribe and monitor medications.

Case Example 2: Elena and the "Hot" Medication

Elena, a 35-year-old Latina woman, was prescribed an antidepressant for persistent depression. After a few weeks, she reported feeling "hot inside" and complained of a persistent dry mouth, leading her to stop taking the medication. The therapist initially suspected side effects but then learned from Elena that she believed the medication was "too hot" for her body, causing an imbalance. This belief was rooted in a traditional Hispanic health system where foods and medicines are categorized as "hot" or "cold" and must be balanced.

The therapist, recognizing this cultural explanatory model, acknowledged Elena's experience. Instead of simply pushing the medication, she explored Elena's concerns. She explained that the medication's side effects, like dry mouth, could indeed make her feel "hot," validating her perception. She then worked with Elena to find ways to "cool" her body while taking the medication, such as drinking specific herbal teas that Elena considered "cooling" or adjusting her diet. The therapist also discussed how different people metabolize medicines differently, and that they could try a different antidepressant that might be less "heating" for her. This culturally informed dialogue helped Elena understand her physical reactions within her own framework and made her willing to try a different medication, which she eventually adhered to successfully.

Case Example 3: The Story of the Adewale Family and Collective Grief

The Adewale family, Nigerian immigrants, sought therapy after their eldest son, a university student, died by suicide. The therapist noted that while the parents expressed profound grief, they also seemed fixated on community rituals and a large, elaborate funeral, frequently saying, "We must do this right for our family and our community." The younger siblings, however, seemed more withdrawn and less inclined to participate in these community expressions. The therapist, trained in individual grief counseling, focused on helping each family member express their personal sadness and process the loss individually.

Despite therapy, the family still seemed stuck in their grief, and the parents expressed frustration that their children weren't "participating in the healing process" enough. The therapist consulted with a colleague who specialized in African cultural contexts. The colleague explained that in many Nigerian cultures, grief is often a collective experience, where the community plays a significant role in mourning rituals, support, and helping the family move forward. Public display of grief, communal feasting, and specific rituals are not just traditions; they are seen as essential steps in the healing process for the entire family and community. Individual withdrawal might be misinterpreted as a lack of respect or proper grieving within this context.

The therapist then shifted her approach. With the family's permission, she attended one of the communal grieving events, observing the powerful role of shared support and ritual. She began to frame therapy in terms of strengthening the family unit to support each other through collective grief, rather than focusing solely on individual sadness. She also explored how the younger siblings might be struggling with the public nature of grief, helping the parents understand their children's different, yet valid, ways of coping within the family's cultural framework. By stepping outside an individualistic lens and embracing the family and community's role in the grieving process, the therapist fostered a more fitting and effective path to healing for the Adewale family.

Chapter 5: Important Points

- **Adaptation is key**: Change therapies to fit the patient's culture, even the main ideas.

- **Mix old and new**: Respectfully include traditional healing ways when they fit and are safe.

- **Family matters**: Understand that for many, family and community are central to care, not just the individual.

- **Medicine needs cultural thought**: Be aware of beliefs about drugs and genetic differences that affect how drugs work.

- **Numbers show it works**: Research proves that culturally adapted interventions are more effective for minority groups.

A Parting Thought

You hold a unique position to offer not just care, but truly connected care. Every person you meet brings their own world with them. By honoring that world—their history, their community, their beliefs—you create a space where genuine healing can begin. It's a journey of continuous learning, and each step you take makes our healing professions stronger and more truly helpful for everyone.

Chapter 6: Immigrant and Refugee Communities

Some groups of people carry stories of resilience and struggle that are distinct from others. We're talking about those who have left their homes, often under very hard conditions, to build new lives elsewhere. Their paths are marked by both hardship and incredible strength. As a mental health professional, understanding their unique challenges and their deep wells of fortitude isn't just helpful—it's essential for providing care that genuinely supports their well-being. This chapter will walk you through the special considerations you'll need when working with immigrant and refugee communities.

Hardships, Moving, and New Culture Stress

People who move to new countries, especially refugees, often face a blend of tough mental health challenges. They might carry deep wounds from **trauma before moving**—from wars, unfair treatment, or violence in their home countries. Then, there's the heavy weight of **displacement**, of being uprooted, and the stress of adapting to a new culture. This is called **acculturative stress**. On top of that, they often deal with unfair treatment and big problems trying to figure out new social rules and health care systems.

This mix of past and present difficulties means their mental health problems are hardly ever simple. Good care needs a **trauma-informed approach** that looks at their whole journey, from where they came from to where they settle. It means knowing about the system problems they face. This approach goes beyond just looking at a person's sickness to include social and system factors. It means you need clear ways to do trauma-informed checks and offer help that accounts for many layers of trauma and stress.

For example, a study found that over 60% of refugees globally have experienced some form of torture or extreme violence before resettlement [23]. Another report stated that rates of PTSD among refugees can be as high as 30-40%, significantly higher than the general population [24]. These numbers underscore the profound impact of pre-migration trauma on these groups. When they arrive in a new country, they often face additional stressors. For instance, in 2023, nearly 85% of asylum seekers in the United Kingdom reported experiencing poverty, which adds another layer of stress and impacts mental well-being [25].

Figuring Out Legal and Social Systems

The complicated rules around legal status, how asylum works, and getting social services really affect the mental health of immigrant and refugee clients, and how much they connect with treatment. Being scared of being sent back, not knowing what will happen in the future, and having trouble understanding confusing official systems can make mental health problems worse. These fears also create big obstacles to getting help. You need to know about these outside pressures and, when it's right, be able to help patients connect with legal help or social support.

Case Example 1: Amina's Fear of the Unknown

Amina, a 28-year-old asylum seeker from Eritrea, was referred to a mental health clinic for severe anxiety and panic attacks. She spoke English fairly well but seemed constantly on edge, often looking over her shoulder and asking about the clock during sessions. She described nightmares about her journey to the US and feared talking about her past in detail. When the therapist suggested working on her trauma, Amina became even more withdrawn.

The therapist, noticing Amina's persistent anxiety about time and her hesitancy to speak about her history, gently asked, "Amina, are there any other worries on your mind, perhaps about your situation here?" Amina then explained, with great hesitation, that her asylum application was pending, and she had an important interview scheduled soon. She was terrified that anything she said in therapy could somehow be used against her, leading to deportation. She also worried about missing deadlines or paperwork. Her anxiety wasn't just about past trauma; it was deeply linked to her precarious legal status.

The therapist, understanding this external stressor, adjusted her approach. She spent time explaining client confidentiality in the US legal system and assured Amina that her therapy notes would not be shared with immigration authorities. With Amina's consent, the therapist connected her to a non-profit legal aid organization specializing in asylum cases. The legal aid group helped Amina understand the process, prepared her for the interview, and clarified legal protections. Knowing her legal situation was being addressed, and feeling that her fears were taken seriously, significantly reduced Amina's general anxiety. This allowed her to feel safer and more ready to begin addressing her past trauma in therapy.

Building Strength and Community Help

Even with big problems, immigrant and refugee communities often show amazing strength. They find power in their culture, their faith, and their community connections. You should look for and use these specific cultural strengths. Working with community groups, cultural associations, and faith-based organizations can give very helpful social support, resources, and a feeling of belonging. These are all crucial for good mental health and fitting in successfully.

Case Example 2: The Garcia Family's Feast

The Garcia family, recently arrived from Guatemala, were struggling to adapt. Mrs. Garcia, who was receiving therapy for depression, mentioned feeling very isolated despite living in a city with a large Latin American population. She missed her family's traditional celebrations and the lively community gatherings she knew back home. The therapist had been trying to connect her with English classes and job support, which were important, but didn't seem to lift her spirits much.

The therapist learned that Mrs. Garcia was a wonderful cook and that traditional meals were a central part of her cultural identity and social connection. She also learned about a local Guatemalan community center that hosted monthly potlucks and cultural events. Instead of just suggesting more formal resources, the therapist encouraged Mrs. Garcia to attend one of the potlucks. She even helped Mrs. Garcia find a recipe for a traditional dish she could bring, framing it as a way to "share her strength and culture."

Mrs. Garcia hesitated at first, but with the therapist's encouragement, she attended. She brought her dish, was warmly welcomed, and instantly felt a connection with others who shared her background. She began attending regularly, making friends, and eventually volunteered to help organize future events. This community connection became a powerful source of resilience, giving her a sense of belonging and purpose. Her depression symptoms lessened significantly as she re-established her cultural community ties. This showed that sometimes, the most effective support comes from helping people tap into their own cultural strengths and community networks.

A Family's Journey in a New Land

Let's think about an immigrant family from a country scarred by war, now seeking mental health support. The parents might show signs of **PTSD** from the trauma they faced before moving, while their children, growing up in a new culture, experience **acculturative stress** and disagreements with their parents due to cultural differences between generations. The family might first talk about physical pains because of cultural rules around expressing problems. A culturally sensitive approach would mean doing a thorough check that includes their history of moving, looking into how they explain sickness, and understanding their family dynamics and cultural values. Help might include trauma-informed therapy for the parents, family therapy to close the gaps between generations, and connecting the family with community support groups that celebrate their culture. This story shows how ideas like trauma, new culture stress, and system problems show up in real life. It also shows how to use culturally sensitive checks and help strategies together.

Case Example 3: The Mohammed Family from Syria

The Mohammed family — parents, adult son, and two teenage daughters — arrived in the U.S. as refugees from Syria, having lived through intense conflict and loss. Mr. Mohammed struggled with nightmares and flashbacks, often withdrawing into himself. Mrs. Mohammed was constantly worried about their safety and the future, expressing her distress through physical aches and pains she called "nerves." Their teenage daughters were quickly learning English and adapting to school, but often clashed with their parents over traditional customs versus American norms. The son, fluent in English, felt caught in the middle, trying to bridge the gap.

Their initial visit to a mental health clinic was difficult. The intake worker focused on individual symptoms and tried to schedule separate appointments for each family member. The family seemed hesitant, especially the parents, who didn't fully explain their past or their cultural ways of expressing pain.

A culturally aware therapist took on the family. First, she scheduled a family meeting, acknowledging that in many Syrian families, decisions and problems are shared. She used a professional Arabic interpreter and started by asking about their journey and what had brought them to America, validating their strength in surviving. She noticed Mr. Mohammed's quietness and Mrs. Mohammed's physical complaints. Instead of pushing for emotional talk right away, she asked, "What do you believe has caused these difficulties for your family since you arrived?"

Mr. Mohammed eventually spoke of his shame at not being able to protect his family and his constant replaying of traumatic events. Mrs. Mohammed explained her "nerves" as her body reacting to constant worry for her children. The daughters talked about feeling torn between their parents' expectations and fitting in at school.

The therapist developed a layered plan:

1. **For the parents**: Individual trauma-focused therapy, but framed in a way that respected their cultural values of family protection and resilience. For Mrs. Mohammed's somatization, the therapist validated her physical pain while gently connecting it to her worries, teaching relaxation techniques that could help both mind and body.

2. **For the daughters**: Support groups for refugee youth, helping them navigate acculturation and intergenerational conflict with peers who understood their experiences.

3. **For the whole family**: Regular family sessions that focused on communication skills, respecting each other's ways of coping, and creating new family traditions that blended Syrian and American elements. The therapist also connected them to a local Syrian community organization that provided cultural events and social support, helping them rebuild a sense of belonging.

This comprehensive approach addressed the varied traumas, acculturative stress, and intergenerational gaps by centering the family's cultural framework and leveraging community resources, leading to a path of healing for everyone.

Chapter 6: Important Points

- **Many layers of hardship**: Immigrants and refugees face severe trauma, displacement, and stress from new cultures.

- **System barriers are real**: Legal worries and social system problems greatly affect mental health and access to care.

- **Strengths count**: These communities have amazing strength from their culture, faith, and community. Use those!

- **Whole person approach**: Care must look at their entire journey and all the outside factors shaping their well-being.

Chapter 7: Indigenous and Traditional Perspectives on Healing

When we talk about healing, it's easy to fall into the trap of thinking there's only one path, typically the one we've been taught. But if you open your mind, you'll find ancient, deep-rooted ways of understanding health and well-being, especially within Indigenous communities. Their histories are etched with pain, but also with incredible endurance and wisdom. This chapter asks you to quiet your assumptions and listen to these powerful, often silenced, voices of healing.

Past Harms and Their Effects Across Generations

Indigenous groups around the world have lived through deep wrongs. These include things like colonialism, being forced to give up their ways, and unfair treatment by systems. These experiences have caused **historical trauma**, which is the total emotional and psychological damage that lasts through many generations, coming from huge group trauma. The effects of things like forced boarding schools or being forced from their lands still show up today in high rates of mental health problems, substance use, and suicide in these communities. Knowing this past is most important for anyone working with Indigenous people.

For example, in Canada, over 150,000 First Nations, Inuit, and Métis children were forced to attend residential schools from the 1800s until 1996 [26]. These schools aimed to "kill the Indian in the child," resulting in widespread abuse, neglect, and the loss of language and culture. Studies show that descendants of residential school survivors have higher rates of depression, anxiety, PTSD, and substance use disorders [27]. Similarly, in the United States, the forced removal of Indigenous peoples from their lands, such as the Cherokee Trail of Tears, led to immense loss and suffering, with psychological impacts still observed today [28]. These events aren't just history; they are living wounds that shape present-day mental health challenges.

Respecting Old Healers and Ceremonies

Old healing ways and spiritual beliefs mean a lot in how many Indigenous cultures approach health and sickness. These ways often involve special gatherings, telling stories, feeling connected to the land, and getting advice from old healers. It's crucial for you, as a Western-trained clinician, to show respect for these ways and, when it's right, work with old healers. If you ignore or dismiss these deeply held beliefs, it can lead to a lack of trust, not following treatment, and poor results. On the other hand, respectfully bringing these beliefs into treatment plans, when appropriate, can greatly help patients connect with care and make the healing relationship stronger. This approach needs careful thought about what fits together and what's fair, making sure that any blending truly helps the patient and respects the truth of the old ways.

Case Example 1: Sarah and the Sweat Lodge

Sarah, a 30-year-old Ojibwe woman, sought therapy for severe anxiety and feelings of hopelessness. She had experienced significant family loss and struggled with intergenerational trauma related to residential schools. In therapy, she made some progress with CBT, but still felt a deep spiritual void. She mentioned to her therapist that her grandmother used to tell stories about the healing power of the **sweat lodge**, and that she felt a pull to reconnect with this traditional ceremony.

The therapist, though unfamiliar with sweat lodges, did not dismiss Sarah's interest. Instead, she asked Sarah to tell her more about what the sweat lodge meant to her. Sarah explained it was a sacred ceremony for cleansing, prayer, and connecting with ancestors and the Creator. She believed it could help her release spiritual burdens. The therapist, respecting Sarah's explanatory model, inquired about how Sarah planned to access a sweat lodge and if there was an elder or traditional helper who could guide her.

With Sarah's permission, the therapist also reached out to an Indigenous cultural consultant associated with their clinic. The consultant explained the importance of the sweat lodge in Ojibwe culture and its potential benefits for holistic healing. The therapist then supported Sarah in finding a reputable community-led sweat lodge ceremony. After attending, Sarah returned to therapy with renewed energy. She described feeling lighter, more connected to her heritage, and better able to cope with her anxiety. She continued therapy, but now felt her spiritual path was also respected, strengthening her trust in the therapist and the overall healing process.

Working Together with Indigenous Communities for Care

Good mental health care for Indigenous communities often means moving past Western models that focus only on the person. Instead, it means using **collaborative care models**. These models put **Indigenous self-determination** first, knowing that communities have the right to decide their own paths to health and healing. They involve projects led by the community, bringing Indigenous knowledge into health care, and creating services that fit the community's values and traditions. Such ways of working build trust and give communities the power to guide their own healing journeys.

Case Example 2: The "Healing Circle" in a Pueblo Community

A community mental health center serving a Pueblo reservation was seeing limited success with individual therapy for young adults struggling with substance use. Many clients would attend a few sessions then stop, citing that it "didn't feel right" or "didn't help the whole family." The clinicians were frustrated by the lack of follow-through.

After consulting with tribal elders and health leaders, the center's director learned that the individualistic approach of Western therapy often conflicted with the Pueblo values of collective well-being and community support. The elders suggested a "Healing Circle" model, led by a respected community elder and co-facilitated by a Western-trained therapist. This circle would meet weekly in a communal space, incorporate storytelling, traditional prayers, and allow for family members to attend and offer support.

The center agreed to try this **collaborative care model**. In the Healing Circle, individuals shared their struggles, but the focus was on how their well-being affected the community and how the community could support their recovery. The elder provided traditional wisdom and guidance, while the therapist offered insights on coping skills, framing them in culturally meaningful ways (e.g., mindfulness as "present moment awareness to the Creator's gifts"). This approach fostered a sense of belonging and collective responsibility that individual therapy had not. Attendance significantly improved, and participants reported feeling more understood and supported. This showed that truly effective care meant letting the community lead and shaping services around their own deep-seated cultural ways.

A Case of Old Beliefs and Healing

Think about a patient from an Indigenous community who talks about feeling down and worried, but says their problems come from a **spiritual imbalance** or a break in harmony with nature, not from a Western diagnosis. They might want to see an old healer or take part in a healing gathering. A culturally skilled clinician would first show they understand and respect the patient's way of explaining their illness. Instead of ignoring their beliefs, the clinician would look into how these old ways might affect how they see sickness and healing. The clinician might then, with the patient's permission, offer to work with an old healer, or support the patient in taking part in cultural gatherings, while also offering Western therapy. This way of working shows how to build trust and strengthen the healing relationship by accepting and using old healing ways, even if they are very different from Western medical ideas.

Case Example 3: Joseph and the Loss of Spirit

Joseph, a 45-year-old Lakota man, came to the clinic with symptoms of severe depression: sadness, loss of appetite, and a deep sense of despair. He told the therapist, "I feel like I've lost my spirit. My connection to the land and my people is broken." His wife added that he had stopped participating in community events and seemed to blame his distress on a recent relocation from the reservation to the city for work.

The therapist, rather than focusing solely on a DSM diagnosis, asked Joseph what "losing his spirit" meant to him and what he believed would help him regain it. Joseph explained that traditional Lakota beliefs hold that disconnection from the land, ceremonies, and community can lead to spiritual illness, which then affects mental and physical health. He spoke of his desire to participate in a Sun Dance ceremony, a sacred ritual that he believed would help him reconnect.

The therapist acknowledged Joseph's explanatory model. She said, "Joseph, it sounds like your spirit is hurting because of this big change in your life, and that connection to your traditions is so important for your healing." She offered to continue traditional talk therapy sessions, focusing on coping strategies for adjusting to city life and processing his grief over the loss of his connection to the land. Crucially, with Joseph's consent, the therapist also helped him connect with an urban Indigenous community center that facilitated traditional ceremonies, including sweat lodges and opportunities to connect with elders. The therapist and Joseph discussed how attending these ceremonies could complement his therapy by addressing his spiritual needs. This dual approach—validating his spiritual explanation while offering Western tools—allowed Joseph to pursue healing that was holistic and culturally meaningful, ultimately leading to a significant improvement in his mood and a renewed sense of purpose.

Key Takeaways:

- **Trauma that lasts**: Indigenous groups carry the heavy load of historical injustices that affect their mental health across generations.

- **Respect old ways**: Acknowledge and, when right, work with traditional healers and ceremonies; they are vital to healing.

- **Community leads**: The best care models for Indigenous communities are led by the community itself, not just Western ideas.

- **Spirit matters**: For many Indigenous people, healing means restoring balance and connection to spirit, land, and community.

Chapter 8: Mental Health for Other Varied Groups

It's time to widen our view even more, isn't it? Cultural understanding isn't just about different countries or skin colors. It stretches to cover many groups, each with their own ways of living and facing life's ups and downs. Whether it's about who you love, how your body works, or what you believe, every person has a distinct social setting that shapes their mental health journey. This chapter asks you to peel back even more layers and learn how to truly tailor your care for all sorts of people.

Customizing Care to Different Cultural and Social Settings

Cultural understanding isn't just about someone's background or nationality; it reaches many other groups with their own cultural and social settings. This includes, but is not limited to, **LGBTQ+ communities, people with disabilities, and specific religious or socioeconomic groups**. Each of these groups might face unique mental health challenges because of societal unfairness, discrimination, or specific life events. For example, LGBTQ+ people might deal with **minority stress**, while people with disabilities might face system barriers to getting help and being included.

It's most important to see how different parts of a person's identity come together, like a queer immigrant or a disabled person of color. These mixing identities can create special experiences of being left out and vulnerable, needing an even more careful and personal way of giving care. You must always keep learning about these different cultural and social settings, actively working against stereotypes, and adjusting your help to fit the specific needs and strengths of each person. This ongoing promise to learn is crucial to avoid making assumptions and to give truly fair and effective care.

For instance, the LGBTQ+ community faces unique stressors. A 2023 survey found that 45% of LGBTQ+ youth in the U.S. seriously considered suicide in the past year, with rates even higher for transgender and nonbinary youth (54%) [29]. This is partly attributed to **minority stress**, which includes experiences of prejudice, discrimination, and the need to hide one's identity. Similarly, individuals with disabilities often experience higher rates of mental health conditions compared to the general population. A 2021 study revealed that adults with disabilities were three times more likely to report having a mental health condition than adults without disabilities [30]. These numbers highlight the urgent need for tailored, informed care.

Case Example 1: Alex, a Nonbinary Teen

Alex, a 16-year-old who identifies as nonbinary and uses "they/them" pronouns, was referred for anxiety and depression. Their parents, while generally supportive, struggled to understand Alex's gender identity and sometimes used incorrect pronouns. At school, Alex faced occasional bullying and felt isolated, worrying about using the "wrong" bathroom or being misgendered by teachers.

The therapist had some basic knowledge about LGBTQ+ issues but realized they needed to go deeper. First, the therapist consistently used Alex's correct pronouns and affirmed Alex's identity. They didn't question Alex's gender, but instead explored what it *meant* for Alex in their daily life. The therapist asked, "Alex, how does being nonbinary affect your anxiety at school?" and "What would help you feel safer and more seen by your family?"

The therapist also helped Alex develop coping strategies for **minority stress**, such as learning how to respond to misgendering or finding supportive online communities. With Alex's consent, the therapist offered to have a family session to help educate Alex's parents. In that session, the therapist explained gender identity in plain terms, using analogies that helped the parents grasp the concept, and guided them on respectful language use. By recognizing and addressing Alex's specific experiences as a nonbinary youth and the related societal pressures, the therapist provided care that was truly relevant and affirming, leading to a significant reduction in Alex's distress.

Case Example 2: Mrs. Rodriguez and Religious Trauma

Mrs. Rodriguez, a 50-year-old woman, sought therapy for severe guilt, panic attacks, and feelings of worthlessness. She identified as a devout Catholic, and initially, the therapist did not explore her religious background beyond noting it in the intake. Mrs. Rodriguez, however, often spoke of "sin" and "punishment" in vague terms.

As therapy progressed, Mrs. Rodriguez became more comfortable. She confessed that her panic attacks began after she left a strict religious community that she now viewed as abusive. She had been taught that questioning authority or leaving the community meant eternal damnation. She felt deep guilt and spiritual despair, believing she was truly "unworthy" and that her mental health problems were divine punishment. This was a case of **religious trauma**.

The therapist, recognizing that Mrs. Rodriguez's distress was deeply intertwined with her religious background, shifted focus. Instead of solely challenging her thoughts as irrational, the therapist acknowledged the real pain of her experience within that community. The therapist helped Mrs. Rodriguez separate genuine spiritual principles from harmful, controlling doctrines. They explored how her prior experiences had weaponized her faith against her, leading to shame and anxiety. The therapist supported Mrs. Rodriguez in finding a more affirming, less rigid spiritual community that aligned with her personal values and helped her reclaim her faith as a source of comfort rather than fear. This culturally sensitive approach, which understood the nuances of religious experience and potential trauma, allowed Mrs. Rodriguez to heal both spiritually and mentally.

Case Example 3: Mr. Davies, a Veteran with a Disability

Mr. Davies, a 40-year-old military veteran, was referred for depression and anger management. He used a wheelchair due to an injury sustained in combat. During initial sessions, he often expressed frustration about accessibility issues in his community and felt his complaints were dismissed by healthcare providers as "just part of his depression." He also felt that his military experience was misunderstood by civilian therapists.

The therapist listened carefully to Mr. Davies's frustrations. She recognized that his disability wasn't just a physical condition; it was a social identity that came with specific barriers and experiences of discrimination. She also understood that his veteran status meant a unique set of cultural norms and potential traumas. Instead of minimizing his complaints about accessibility, she validated them, saying, "It sounds incredibly frustrating to deal with those barriers. Your anger makes sense."

The therapist helped Mr. Davies connect with local veteran support groups, where he could share his experiences with others who understood the unique challenges of military life and living with a combat-related disability. She also worked with him to advocate for better accessibility in his community, turning his anger into empowered action. When discussing his combat trauma, she used language that resonated with his military background, focusing on concepts like "mission," "comradeship," and "reintegration." By acknowledging his disability as a social factor and his veteran status as a distinct cultural group, the therapist created a space where Mr. Davies felt truly heard and understood, leading to significant improvements in his mood and coping skills.

Key Points

- **Culture is broad**: Cultural understanding applies to LGBTQ+ people, those with disabilities, various religious groups, and people of different social standings.

- **Identities overlap**: Recognize that people often have many identities that can cause unique experiences of hardship.

- **Address unfairness**: These groups often face unique mental health challenges from societal unfairness and discrimination.

- **Keep learning**: Always challenge your own assumptions and tailor care to the specific needs and strengths of each person.

- **Numbers show disparities**: Statistics reveal higher rates of mental health struggles in marginalized communities, showing a clear need for custom care.

Chapter 9: Navigating Ethical Puzzles in Diverse Care

Ethical Guideposts in Culturally Rich Care

In our line of work, we all have a set of clear principles that light our way. We aim to **do good** (beneficence), to **avoid harm** (non-maleficence), to **respect choices** (autonomy), to **be fair** (justice), to **keep promises** (fidelity), and to **be truthful** (veracity). These aren't just fancy words; they're the very foundation of trusting relationships in care.

But here's where it gets interesting: what seems like "doing good" in one culture might look very different in another. Or, what "respecting choices" means for an individual might clash with how a family makes decisions together. This is where cultural setting can truly change how these duties are understood or how much weight they carry. For instance, in a highly individualistic society, a patient's personal choice might be seen as the ultimate good. But in a more collectivistic culture, the well-being and honor of the family might take precedence over individual desires. Your task is to understand these different viewpoints, not judge them.

This brings us to the idea of "**ethical humility**"—it's simply knowing when you don't know, and having the good sense to ask for help. No one expects you to have all the answers for every culture and every situation. The strength comes in recognizing your limits, staying curious, and reaching out for guidance when you face a new ethical twist. This active stance means you are always learning and growing, which directly helps the people you serve.

When Traditions Meet Modern Practice: Finding Common Ground

Sometimes, the ways people have always healed and the modern practices we use can feel like they're on different planets. This creates dilemmas around **traditional healing practices** that might seem to conflict with evidence-based care. Think about herbal remedies that a patient relies on, or spiritual rituals they believe are essential for their well-being. Your job isn't to dismiss these; it's to understand their meaning and, if possible, find a way for them to coexist safely with Western methods.

You'll also run into cultural norms around sensitive topics. Imagine a young person talking about **self-harm disclosures** in a culture where such an admission might bring great shame to the family. Or consider **issues of honor**, where a patient's actions might be viewed through a community lens that values reputation above individual expression. You might even encounter discussions around **forced marriages** or practices like **female genital cutting (FGC)**, where deeply ingrained cultural traditions clash dramatically with Western ethical and legal standards of human rights and safety. In such situations, it's not about quick judgments but about careful navigation.

The goal is always to find respectful ways to bring different approaches together or to explain them so that you don't make a patient feel like their beliefs are wrong. It's about building bridges, not walls. You might say, "I understand that [traditional practice] is very meaningful to you. Let's talk about how we can make sure it works safely alongside the care we offer here," rather than, "That's not science-based; you should stop it."

Case Example 1: Elena and the "Evil Eye"

Elena, a 19-year-old Latina woman, was being treated for anxiety and recurring nightmares. During a session, she quietly confessed that she believed her problems were caused by *mal de ojo* (the "evil eye") cast upon her by a jealous relative. She had consulted a traditional curandera (healer) who performed a ritual to cleanse her aura and given her specific amulets to wear. Elena felt some relief from the curandera's help and planned to continue seeing her.

The therapist, trained in cognitive behavioral therapy, initially felt a conflict. Her scientific training emphasized empirical evidence, and the concept of an "evil eye" seemed at odds with psychological principles. However, she remembered the importance of respecting explanatory models. Instead of challenging Elena's belief directly, she asked, "Elena, you feel relief from the curandera's work. What do you believe the 'evil eye' does, and how does her healing help you?"

Elena explained that the curandera's ritual made her feel protected and restored her spiritual balance, which in turn helped her feel less anxious. The therapist realized that while she didn't share the belief, the *process* of feeling protected and restoring balance was therapeutically helpful for Elena. The therapist framed their therapy as complementary: "It sounds like the curandera helps you with the spiritual protection you need, and here, we can work on skills for managing the worries that still come up and helping you sleep better. Perhaps they can both help you feel stronger." By finding a common language and respecting Elena's traditional healing, the therapist avoided a clash and maintained a trusting relationship, allowing Elena to benefit from both approaches.

Privacy and the Family Circle: Who Needs to Know?

One of the trickiest areas often involves **privacy and how much family should be involved**. Your professional rules usually emphasize individual privacy and confidentiality. But in many cultures, the idea of an individual's private life, separate from their family, just isn't the main way things work. **Family and community involvement** are central.

You'll find situations where family members expect to be part of treatment decisions or want to know everything that's going on. In some collectivistic cultures, a diagnosis of mental illness might be seen as a family issue, not just an individual one, and decisions are often made by elders or the whole group.

So, how do you **balance patient confidentiality with family needs and safety**, especially when working with minors or vulnerable adults? It requires thoughtful steps:

1. **Understand the cultural norm**: Ask the patient (and respectfully, the family) about their views on privacy and

family involvement. "In your family, how are serious personal matters usually discussed? Who is typically involved in making health decisions?"

2. **Explain your rules clearly**: Describe your clinic's confidentiality policies in a way that respects their culture, if possible. "In my work, I promise to keep what you tell me private, unless you give me permission to share. How do you feel about that in your family?"

3. **Get informed consent for family involvement**: If family involvement is culturally expected and helpful for the patient, always get the patient's clear permission about what can be shared and with whom. This could involve a written consent form, or a clear verbal agreement witnessed by all parties.

4. **Define boundaries together**: Help the patient decide what they *want* to share with their family and what they want to keep private.

5. **Use it as a strength**: If family involvement is appropriate, view it as a source of support, not just a challenge.

Case Example 2: The Family's "Secret" and Confidentiality

Jamal, a 16-year-old immigrant from a conservative Middle Eastern country, was struggling with depression and suicidal thoughts. He confided in his therapist about deep family conflicts, including a strained relationship with his strict father who had very traditional expectations for him. Jamal pleaded with the therapist not to tell his parents about his suicidal thoughts, fearing severe punishment or being sent back to his home country.

The therapist faced a clear ethical dilemma: her duty to protect Jamal from harm versus her promise of confidentiality, which Jamal deeply valued given his cultural context. She knew that in Jamal's culture, family authority was paramount, and mental health issues were often kept secret to maintain family honor. Directly breaking confidentiality might lead to Jamal being pulled from therapy entirely, and potentially facing harsh repercussions at home, which could put him at greater risk.

The therapist consulted with a cultural expert familiar with Jamal's background and also sought clinical supervision. They discussed the nuance of family involvement in Jamal's culture and the specific risks he perceived. The supervisor suggested working *with* Jamal to identify a trusted family member (perhaps an aunt or an elder) who could be brought into the conversation in a controlled way, or to help Jamal find a way to communicate a *limited* amount of information to his parents that would alleviate their immediate concerns without disclosing everything. The therapist explained to Jamal her duty to ensure his safety, but also her commitment to respecting his family's values. Together, they planned how to tell his father that Jamal was "having a hard time with the pressure of school and adapting to the new country" (a more culturally acceptable explanation) and that he needed support. This allowed Jamal to feel some control, while still addressing the safety concerns indirectly and with his buy-in. It was a careful balance, but one that preserved the therapeutic relationship and potentially kept Jamal safer.

Power and Privilege in the Healing Room: Seeing Yourself Clearly

As a clinician, you hold a certain power. You have knowledge, a title, and control over the session space. You also bring your own background—your race, gender, social class, education—into the room. This means you need to be aware of how your own **position (of power, privilege, or a specific cultural background) can affect the therapeutic relationship**. For instance, if you are a White, middle-class therapist working with a refugee from a non-Western country, there's an inherent power imbalance that might make the patient hesitant to speak freely or challenge your ideas.

You'll also need to address situations where a patient might:

- **Defer too much**: They might agree with everything you say out of respect for your position, even if they don't truly understand or agree.

- **Distrust you**: Due to past bad experiences with systems of power (e.g., healthcare discrimination, government authorities), a patient from a marginalized group might approach you with suspicion.

Your role is to **use your position responsibly to advocate for the patient**. This means creating a safe space where they feel empowered to speak, questioning their deference gently, and working actively to build trust by showing genuine humility and respect for their experiences. It means recognizing your own blind spots and actively seeking to understand how your own background might influence your assumptions about the patient.

Case Example 3: Dr. Evans and the Reluctant Elder

Dr. Evans, a highly educated, young, male psychiatrist, was consulting on the case of an elderly Indigenous man, Mr. Bear, who was experiencing severe depression following the loss of his wife. Mr. Bear was quiet in sessions, often looking down, and would give very brief answers to Dr. Evans' direct questions about his symptoms or feelings. Dr. Evans felt frustrated by what he perceived as Mr. Bear's "lack of engagement."

Dr. Evans later realized that his own position—young, male, non-Indigenous, and highly educated—could be impacting Mr. Bear's behavior. In many Indigenous cultures, respect for elders is paramount, and it might be seen as inappropriate for a younger person to ask direct, personal questions of an elder, especially about emotional pain. Avoiding eye contact could also be a sign of respect, not disinterest.

Dr. Evans adjusted his approach. He consulted with an Indigenous elder from the local community (with Mr. Bear's permission). The elder explained the cultural norms of communication and respect. In the next session, Dr. Evans consciously lowered his gaze more often, spoke more softly, and began the session by sharing a little more about himself, as a way of building relationship. He shifted from direct questions about symptoms to open-ended invitations like, "Mr. Bear, if you feel comfortable, I'm here to listen to your story. What has been on your heart since your wife passed?" He also asked about Mr. Bear's community and family, showing respect for his relational world. Slowly, Mr. Bear began to share more, not because his symptoms changed, but because Dr. Evans recognized and adapted to the power dynamics and cultural expectations in the room, making Mr. Bear feel respected and safe.

Handling the Stress of Ethical Challenges

Let's be real: wrestling with these complex ethical puzzles can take a toll on you. The **emotional weight of grappling with complex ethical dilemmas** is no small thing. You might experience **moral distress**—that feeling of knowing the right thing to do but being unable to do it due to external constraints—or **fatigue** from constantly balancing competing values. This is part of the work, but it's not something you should carry alone.

It's vital to have strategies for managing this stress. Sometimes it's about acknowledging the limits of what you can control, and other times it's about finding the courage to advocate for a solution. Knowing when to step back, get some fresh air, or talk it out with a trusted colleague is just as important as knowing your ethical principles.

Steps to Solve Culturally Complex Ethical Problems

When you find yourself facing an ethical puzzle that has a cultural twist, here's a simple, actionable framework to help you navigate:

1. **Identify the Core Dilemma**: What are the competing values or principles at stake? (e.g., individual autonomy vs. family cohesion, beneficence vs. cultural practice).

2. **Gather Cultural Information**: What are the patient's and family's explanatory models, beliefs, and practices related to the issue? What are the cultural norms around communication, decision-making, and privacy? *This is where cultural humility shines.*

3. **Consult Widely**: Talk to supervisors, ethical committees, and, most importantly, **cultural consultants or community elders** who can offer a culturally informed perspective. They can help you understand the nuances you might be missing.

4. **Brainstorm Solutions**: Generate as many possible solutions as you can, even those that seem unlikely at first. Think outside your usual Western frameworks.

5. **Evaluate Solutions Against Principles (and Cultural Context)**: Which solutions best uphold ethical principles *while also* respecting the patient's cultural context and minimizing harm? Consider the potential consequences of each option from the patient's cultural viewpoint.

6. **Seek Patient/Family Input**: Discuss the options openly with the patient and, if appropriate and consented, their family. Work collaboratively to find a solution that feels respectful and workable for them.

7. **Act and Review**: Put the chosen solution into action and regularly check in to see if it's working and if any new ethical questions arise.

This framework isn't a magic wand, but it provides a clear path forward when the waters get choppy. The importance of **consultation** cannot be overstated here—talking to someone who has walked this path before, or someone who holds deep knowledge of a specific culture, is your best friend when you're stuck.

Summary:

- **Ethics meets culture**: Your core ethical duties must be understood and applied with cultural awareness.

- **Traditional ways count**: Learn to respectfully approach traditional healing and sensitive cultural practices.

- **Privacy is layered**: Understand varied cultural views on privacy and how family involvement fits in.

- **Know your own power**: See how your own position affects the patient relationship and use it responsibly.

- **Don't go it alone**: Ethical dilemmas are tough; use supervisors and cultural consultants to help you through.

- **Framework for choices**: Follow clear steps to make ethical decisions in culturally complex situations.

Chapter 10: Self-Care for the Culturally Wise Clinician

The Weight of Caring: Understanding Empathic Strain

Working with people from many different backgrounds, especially those who've gone through trauma or unfair treatment, can carry a heavy emotional load. It's not just about listening to their stories; it's about feeling some of their pain, too. This is what we call **empathic strain** or **compassion fatigue** [39]. It's that feeling of being worn out because you've poured so much of your emotion into helping others.

Think about it: you're bearing witness to systemic injustices, hearing firsthand accounts of discrimination, displacement, and historical trauma. These aren't just abstract ideas; they're the lived experiences of the people sitting across from you. This can take a unique toll, making you feel sad, frustrated, or even angry about the unfairness in the world. Recognizing this emotional weight isn't a sign of weakness; it's a sign that you're paying attention and that your heart is in the work.

Case Example 1: Dr. Ben Carter and the Weight of Injustice

Dr. Ben Carter, a therapist working in a community clinic, often served clients who were refugees from various war-torn regions. He prided himself on his cultural humility and trauma-informed approach. However, after a particularly intense week of sessions—including one client who recounted horrific acts of violence and another who detailed years of systemic discrimination in their new country—Dr. Carter found himself unusually irritable at home. He had trouble sleeping, replayed client stories in his head, and felt a sense of hopelessness about the world's problems. He was showing signs of **empathic strain**.

During his supervision session, Dr. Carter admitted, "I feel like I'm carrying all their burdens. I know I can't fix global injustices, but it's just so heavy to hear it week after week." His supervisor, recognizing the signs of compassion fatigue, didn't dismiss his feelings. Instead, she validated them: "Ben, that's a very real feeling. You're hearing about profound suffering and systemic issues, and it's natural to feel that weight. It means you're truly connecting with your clients."

The supervisor then helped Dr. Carter understand that while empathy is good, excessive absorption of client distress can be harmful. She suggested strategies to create more emotional distance while still providing compassionate care. This included specific "detaching" rituals after sessions (e.g., taking a walk, listening to music), consciously leaving work at the office, and focusing on the small wins and resilience of his clients, rather than solely on their suffering. Understanding the source of his fatigue helped Dr. Carter develop tailored coping strategies.

Simple Ways to Recharge Your Own Battery

Just like your phone needs to charge, so do you. Ignoring this leads to a dead battery, and then you can't help anyone. These are practical **self-care strategies** that aren't fluffy or complicated; they're essential parts of your professional practice.

- **Setting boundaries**: This is huge. It means having clear lines between your work and your personal life. Don't check work emails at midnight. Don't let sessions run over constantly. Your time off is truly *off*.

- **Mindfulness**: Even a few minutes a day of simply paying attention to your breath, your senses, or the moment can calm a busy mind. This helps you stay present with your clients without getting lost in their distress.

- **Hobbies**: Have something you love doing that has absolutely nothing to do with mental health. Whether it's gardening, painting, playing an instrument, or building model ships, it's your brain's reset button.

- **Time in nature**: Getting outside, even for a short walk, can surprisingly refresh your outlook.

- **Physical health**: Don't underestimate sleep, good food, and moving your body. These are the basic building blocks of energy and resilience. If you're running on fumes, your empathy will drain faster.

These small, everyday practices can make a very big difference in how much energy you have to keep going. They aren't selfish; they're what allow you to continue giving.

Building Your Own Crew: Mentors, Peers, and Support Groups

Trying to do this work alone is a recipe for getting worn out. A strong **support network** isn't a luxury; it's a must. You need people who understand the unique challenges of cultural work.

- **Finding mentors**: Look for experienced professionals who have been doing culturally sensitive work for a while. They can offer advice, share their own struggles, and give you perspective when you feel lost.

- **The power of peer supervision and consultation groups**: These are spaces where you can talk about tough cases with colleagues who are also trying to be culturally aware. You can share feelings, get different ideas, and offer support to each other. It's a place to say, "I'm not sure how to handle this culturally, what do you all think?"

- **Connecting with cultural consultants**: Sometimes, you need specific knowledge. Having access to cultural consultants or community elders—people from the culture your patient belongs to—can be invaluable for your own learning and for understanding a situation more deeply. They can help you see blind spots you didn't even know you had.

Case Example 2: The Therapist's Peer Support Group

Sarah, a therapist who had been practicing for five years, recently moved to a new city with a much more diverse population than she was used to. She found herself feeling uncertain about some of her cases, particularly those involving traditions she knew little about. She was worried about making mistakes or offending clients. She realized she was isolating herself and starting to feel overwhelmed.

Sarah sought out a local peer supervision group focused on multicultural practice. In her first meeting, she presented a case about a patient who was hesitant to make eye contact and seemed to agree with everything she said, making Sarah question if the patient was truly engaged. Other therapists in the group, some with more experience in collectivist cultures, immediately offered insights. "That's common in cultures that value respect for authority," one said. "It's not disinterest; it's often a sign of deference. You might try observing their non-verbal cues more, or asking open-ended questions that invite a narrative rather than a direct answer."

This peer feedback was a game-changer for Sarah. She realized her own assumptions about "engagement" were culturally bound. The group became a safe space where she could openly share her uncertainties without judgment, learn from others' experiences, and process her own discomfort. This network of support directly reduced her stress and increased her confidence in her culturally sensitive practice.

Avoiding Being Worn Out by Cultural Work

It's one thing to understand burnout; it's another to avoid it. **Spotting the early signs of burnout** specific to culturally challenging cases is key. Are you feeling more cynical about your work? Are you less excited to see certain clients? Do you feel like you're constantly fighting an uphill battle against systemic issues? These could be red flags.

You need **strategies for managing caseloads and preventing overload**. This means being realistic about how many clients you can truly serve effectively, especially if many of them have complex cultural needs. Sometimes, it means **learning to say "no"** to new referrals or advocating for smaller caseloads if your clinic is stretching you too thin. It's also about **setting realistic expectations for yourself**. You can't be an expert in every culture, and you can't fix every societal problem. Your goal is to be helpful and respectful within your scope.

Learning Continues: Beyond the Classroom

Cultural understanding isn't a degree you earn and then put on a shelf. It's a lifelong process, and it needs to become a **sustainable habit** for you.

- **Engaging in personal cultural immersion experiences respectfully**: This doesn't mean becoming an anthropologist. It means actively seeking out opportunities to learn about other cultures in respectful ways—attending cultural festivals, visiting community centers, trying new cuisines, or engaging in conversations with people from different backgrounds. Always approach these as a learner, not an expert.

- **Reading widely, consuming diverse media, and seeking out new perspectives**: Beyond academic journals, read novels, watch films, listen to music, and follow news sources from different parts of the world. This helps broaden your understanding in ways textbooks can't.

- **Reflecting on your own cultural journey and how it changes over time**: Your own cultural identity isn't static. As you grow and learn, your own understanding of yourself and your place in the world changes, too. Regularly thinking about this personal journey helps you better understand the experiences of others.

Staying Strong and Never Giving Up on Fairness

This work can sometimes feel like trying to move mountains with a spoon. You're trying to help individuals, but you constantly see the bigger problems—the systemic injustices, the deep-rooted inequalities. It's easy to get discouraged.

But here's why your self-care matters so much: it's how you **connect your personal well-being to your role as an advocate for systemic change**. If you're burnt out, you can't be an effective voice. Taking care of yourself means you have the energy and clarity to push for those bigger changes.

Find ways to **find joy and meaning in the work to sustain your passion**. Celebrate the small victories, the moments of connection, the patient who finally feels heard. These are the fuel for the long game. Because cultural change is slow. It takes persistence. It takes many, many people, working little by little, to shift things. Your commitment, fueled by your own well-being, is a crucial part of that grand, necessary effort.

Chapter 12: Important Points

- **Know the emotional cost**: Working with diverse populations, especially those with trauma, can lead to empathic strain and compassion fatigue.

- **Charge your battery**: Use practical self-care like boundaries, mindfulness, hobbies, and physical health to maintain your energy.

- **Build your support team**: Mentors, peer groups, and cultural consultants are essential for guidance and emotional backup.

- **Watch for burnout signs**: Be aware of the signals that you're getting worn out and take steps to manage your workload and expectations.

- **Learning is a life habit**: Continuously seek new knowledge and experiences about diverse cultures, personally and professionally.

- **Stay strong for change**: Your self-care allows you to keep fighting for fairness and contribute to bigger systemic improvements.

Chapter 11: Self-Reflection and Finding Your Blind Spots

Spotting Your Own Biases and What You Assume

A true mark of cultural skill is your ability to truly look at yourself and find your own hidden biases and assumptions. These unconscious biases can really mess with your professional judgment and the care you give. They can lead to wrong diagnoses, treatments that do not work, and keep health problems unequal. This means that dealing with your own biases isn't just a nice thing to do; it's a must for keeping patients safe and giving fair care.

You have to constantly look at yourself to see your own limits and biases. This active looking can be helped by things like writing in a journal, taking certain tests that show hidden biases, or carefully going over past cases where you worked with patients. By understanding that cultural understanding is a path of constant learning and humility, you can change self-reflection from just a passive idea into a real, active skill that directly helps your patients. This ongoing promise is very important for reducing the harmful effects of bias in your work.

For example, a study using the Implicit Association Test (IAT) found that a large percentage of healthcare providers hold **implicit biases** against racial and ethnic minorities [31]. These biases, even if not conscious, can affect clinical decisions, such as pain management. Research shows that Black patients are significantly less likely to receive appropriate pain medication compared to White patients, partly due to implicit biases that Black individuals have a higher pain tolerance [32]. This demonstrates how unchecked biases can lead to tangible disparities in care.

Growing in Cultural Humility and Learning Always

As we've talked about, cultural humility isn't a place you get to; it's a constant journey. It means promising to always look at yourself and keep learning. Ways to grow in this include:

- **Looking for different viewpoints**: Actively seek out books, movies, news, and personal stories from many different cultures. This helps you see the world through other people's eyes.

- **Getting to know other cultures**: If possible, spend time in diverse communities. This isn't about becoming an expert, but about experiencing other ways of life firsthand, respectfully.

- **Staying up-to-date**: Keep up with new research and the best ways to provide care that respects culture. The world changes, and so should your knowledge.

This constant effort makes sure that you stay flexible and can respond well to the changing needs of all sorts of people.

Dealing with Small Insults and Unfair Treatment in Your Work

You must be ready to spot and handle **microaggressions** effectively. These are small, often unintentional, ways people show prejudice. They might come from others towards your patients, or even, without meaning to, from you as a clinician. To create a safe and welcoming space for healing, you need to actively challenge unfair comments or actions. You must also show patients that you hear and believe their experiences of unfair treatment, making sure they feel seen, heard, and respected no matter their background.

Case Example 1: The "Exotic" Patient

A new therapist, eager to show cultural interest, met a patient, Ms. Tran, who was from Vietnam. During their first session, the therapist, meaning to be friendly, said, "Oh, your culture is so exotic! Do you still practice those ancient rituals?" Ms. Tran politely smiled, but inside, she felt a little uncomfortable. She sensed the therapist saw her as different and perhaps a curiosity, rather than just a person seeking help. She then became less open in subsequent sessions.

The therapist, later reviewing her notes and feeling a slight disconnect, discussed the interaction in supervision. Her supervisor gently pointed out that while the therapist meant well, the word "exotic" can make someone feel like an outsider or a spectacle. It implies a sense of "otherness" rather than shared humanity. It was a **microaggression**, subtle but impactful. The supervisor suggested that instead of making assumptions or using broad, potentially demeaning terms, the therapist could simply ask, "What aspects of your background or culture are most important to you?"

In the next session, the therapist apologized. "Ms. Tran," she said, "I wanted to apologize if my comment about your culture being 'exotic' made you feel uncomfortable. My intention was to show interest, but I realize my words might have made you feel like an outsider, and that's not what I want. I'm here to learn from you." Ms. Tran seemed surprised but relieved. She then shared that she appreciated the apology and felt more comfortable. This open apology, born from self-reflection and recognizing the impact of a microaggression, rebuilt trust and opened the door for Ms. Tran to share more freely about her true struggles and how her cultural background influenced them.

Help from Others and Peer Support in Varied Settings

The complexities of working with many different cultures mean it's very important to get regular help from supervisors and talk with other professionals. These settings give you great chances to:

- **Go over hard cases**: Talk through difficult situations with patients and get advice.

- **Look at your own reactions**: Explore your feelings and biases that might come up during sessions.

- **Spot what you don't see**: Get help seeing your own blind spots that might affect your work.

- **Get advice**: Learn from experienced colleagues.

These kinds of support systems are crucial for growing in your profession and for keeping your work ethical and effective in varied cultural settings.

Case Example 2: The Therapist's Unspoken Frustration

A therapist was working with a young man from a collectivistic culture who consistently brought his mother to therapy sessions. The therapist, trained in individual therapy where autonomy is emphasized, felt frustrated that the mother would often answer questions for the son or interrupt him, hindering what the therapist saw as the son's individual progress. The therapist started to feel impatient in sessions, though she tried to hide it.

During peer supervision, the therapist described the situation, expressing her frustration. A more experienced colleague, who had worked with many families from collectivistic backgrounds, offered a different viewpoint. "It sounds like you're feeling a pull to the individual model," she said, "but in some cultures, the family *is* the unit of care. The mother might see her role as protecting her son, or helping him express himself in a way that respects family honor. Her presence isn't necessarily resistance; it's cultural support."

The supervisor suggested that instead of seeing the mother as an obstacle, the therapist could explore her role and perhaps even use her presence as a resource. "Have you tried asking the mother, 'What are your hopes for your son from these sessions?' or 'How does your family usually help each other with these kinds of problems?'" she suggested. This peer input helped the therapist reframe her perspective. She realized her frustration stemmed from her own cultural lens about individualism. In the next session, she changed her approach, engaging the mother more directly and respectfully, which unexpectedly opened up the son, who then felt more comfortable sharing, knowing his mother was part of the process.

Case Example 3: Addressing Bias in Case Presentation

During a team case conference, a clinician was presenting a case of a patient from a low-income background who was struggling with adherence to medication for a mood disorder. The clinician repeatedly used phrases like, "She just doesn't seem motivated enough," and "It's hard to reach her, she lives in a tough neighborhood." While not overtly discriminatory, some team members noticed a subtle tone of frustration that seemed to attribute the patient's challenges to her circumstances rather than looking at systemic barriers or the patient's strengths.

Another supervisor in the room, practicing cultural humility, gently interrupted the presentation. "Thank you for sharing, that sounds like a really tough situation for both you and the patient," they started. "When we hear about challenges with motivation or access, sometimes our own experiences or assumptions can color how we describe the situation. Could we explore what external factors might be making adherence hard for her, like transportation, childcare, or the cost of medication? And what strengths do you see in her, despite these challenges?"

This intervention, a direct but kind challenge to a potentially biased framing, shifted the team's discussion. The clinician reflected and realized she had indeed focused on the patient's perceived shortcomings rather than the systemic hurdles. The team then brainstormed concrete solutions, such as connecting the patient to a community health worker who could assist with transportation and medication costs, and exploring ways to frame medication adherence that fit her life better. This example shows how supervisors and peers can actively spot and correct subtle biases, turning a potentially negative bias into an opportunity for more effective and equitable care.

Chapter 9: Important Points

- **Look within**: Your ability to find and face your own hidden biases is a cornerstone of good care.

- **Always learn**: Cultural humility means you commit to constantly evaluating yourself and seeking new knowledge.

- **Speak up**: Be ready to spot and deal with subtle insults or unfair treatment, whether from others or yourself.

- **Get help**: Supervision and peer talks are must-haves for handling tough cases and growing professionally in varied settings.

- **Bias impacts care**: Unchecked biases can lead to real problems, like unfair treatment and worse outcomes for patients.

Chapter 12: Building a Culturally Skilled Practice and System

You've learned to look inward, to reflect on your own journey, and to sharpen your skills in the room with a patient. But here's the thing: individual effort, however strong, can only do so much when the very ground we stand on—our healthcare systems—isn't always built for everyone. This last chapter is your call to action, reminding you that your role doesn't stop at the clinic door. You have a voice, and it's a powerful one, especially when it comes to pushing for changes that make care fairer for all.

Speaking Up for System Changes and New Rules

While your own cultural skill is super important, it's not enough to fix all the big health differences we see in mental health care. People from different racial and ethnic groups often face big gaps in care because of many system problems. Also, people who have moved to new countries or are refugees often have trouble dealing with new social and health care systems. These observations show that the problem is deeply rooted in how systems are set up. This means your individual skill, while needed, can't solve the whole problem alone.

Because you work directly with patients and see these problems firsthand, you are in a special spot to speak up for bigger system and policy changes in your workplace, health care systems, and society at large. This means that a culturally skilled clinician does more than just work in a therapy room; they also actively help shape fairer health care systems. So, this guide encourages you to see yourself as someone who can make a difference, offering advice on how to speak up effectively to get rid of system problems and help everyone get fair access to good care.

For instance, national data shows significant disparities in mental healthcare access and outcomes. For example, in the U.S., only 33% of Black adults with a mental illness receive mental health services, compared to 52% of White adults [33]. Among Asian Americans, the rate is even lower, at just 20% [34]. These disparities are not just about individual choices; they reflect systemic barriers like lack of culturally matched providers, language access issues, and historical mistrust of the healthcare system. Another example: a 2022 report highlighted that only 4.7% of psychologists in the U.S. are Black, and even fewer, 1.9%, are Asian, highlighting a stark lack of diversity among providers [35]. These statistics underline the urgent need for systemic changes in training, recruitment, and policy to build a workforce and system that truly reflects and serves the diversity of our communities.

Continuing Your Learning and Growing as a Professional

The world of cultural variety is always changing. This means you need to keep learning and growing professionally. This includes taking part in special training, workshops, and studying on your own to make your knowledge deeper and your cultural skills sharper. Staying up-to-date with new research and the best ways to provide care makes sure you can offer the most current and helpful services.

Case Example 1: The Clinic's Cultural Audit

A mental health clinic, noticing that their patient population was becoming increasingly diverse but their staff remained largely homogenous, decided to conduct a **cultural audit**. This meant looking at their intake forms, waiting room materials, outreach strategies, and even the cultural diversity of their therapeutic approaches. They found that their forms used primarily Western terms, their waiting room lacked diverse language materials, and their outreach was not reaching key immigrant communities.

A culturally competent clinician on staff volunteered to lead a committee to address these issues. They worked to:

- **Revise intake forms**: Adding questions about cultural identity, spiritual beliefs, and preferred language/interpreter needs.

- **Diversify materials**: Ensuring brochures and signs were in multiple languages, and that images reflected the diversity of the community.

- **Community outreach**: Partnering with local cultural centers and faith-based organizations to host informational sessions.

- **Staff training**: Organizing regular cultural competence training sessions, bringing in speakers from diverse community groups to share their perspectives.

This systemic effort, driven by internal advocacy, resulted in a significant increase in trust from diverse communities and improved patient engagement, showing how small changes at a system level can have a big impact.

What's Next for Cultural Understanding in Care

The field of cultural understanding in mental health is always moving forward, with new research always looking for fresh ideas. What's coming next includes putting cultural understanding into online mental health tools, dealing with mental health problems around the world, and making more detailed ways to look at how different parts of a person's identity come together. You are encouraged to help this growing body of knowledge and practice, sharing your experiences and ideas to help the field move forward and make care better for everyone.

Case Example 2: Developing a Culturally Adapted Digital Tool

A tech company was developing a new app for anxiety management, based on Cognitive Behavioral Therapy (CBT) principles. An initial trial showed that while it was effective for some users, it had lower engagement rates among Asian American users. A culturally competent mental health professional was brought in as a consultant.

Upon review, the consultant identified several issues:

- The app's examples of stressful situations were very individualistic (e.g., "My boss criticized my work"), which didn't resonate with users from collectivistic cultures where family honor or community standing might be greater stressors.

- The language used was direct and confrontational in challenging negative thoughts, which could feel disrespectful in cultures that value indirect communication or harmony.

- There were no options to include family members in the coping strategies.

The consultant recommended **cultural adaptation** for the app:

- **Adding diverse scenarios**: Including examples related to family expectations, community pressure, or intergenerational conflict.

- **Adjusting language**: Softening the tone of cognitive restructuring prompts to be more inquisitive and less directive.

- **Including family modules**: Creating optional sections where users could learn how to discuss anxiety with family members or seek support within their family unit.

After these adaptations, a second trial showed significantly increased engagement and effectiveness among Asian American users. This shows how cultural understanding can be woven into new technologies to serve diverse populations better.

Case Example 3: Advocating for Language Access in a Hospital System

A large hospital system, facing an increasing number of patients with limited English proficiency, was experiencing communication breakdowns and patient complaints. Interpreters were often unavailable, leading to reliance on family members or untrained staff, especially in mental health emergencies.

A group of nurses and therapists, recognizing the direct impact on patient safety and quality of care, formed a task force. They gathered data on the number of non-English speaking patients, the frequency of interpreter requests, and adverse events linked to communication errors. They then presented their findings to hospital administration, advocating for a **system-wide policy change** to prioritize professional medical interpreters.

Their advocacy efforts included:

- **Presenting compelling statistics**: Highlighting the risk of misdiagnosis and poor outcomes when professional interpreters aren't used.

- **Proposing clear guidelines**: Suggesting a policy mandating professional interpreter use for all clinical encounters where a language barrier exists.

- **Recommending budget allocation**: Showing how an investment in interpreters could reduce readmissions, improve patient satisfaction, and decrease legal risks.

- **Developing a training program**: Offering to train staff on effective interpreter use.

As a result of their persistent and data-driven advocacy, the hospital system implemented a new policy, invested in more professional interpreters (both in-person and telehealth), and created a mandatory training program for all clinical staff. This demonstrates how individual clinicians, working together, can push for and achieve significant systemic change that benefits thousands of patients.

Conclusion

The need for cultural understanding in mental health care is clear. It's driven by our increasingly varied societies and the unfair health problems that simply won't go away. This guide has given you a full picture, starting with basic ideas about culture and identity, and moving to hands-on skills for checking, talking, and changing how you help. It has stressed the big impact of cultural factors on mental health experiences and the absolutely crucial role of cultural humility as a path of constant looking inward and learning.

Key points throughout this guide show that cultural understanding isn't just an extra skill; it's a fundamental requirement for care that is morally right, works well, and is fair. The shift towards cultural humility means a deeper promise to fix power differences and create helping relationships where everyone works together. Knowing that health problems come from many levels of system issues means you, as a clinician, are not just a direct caregiver but also a very important voice for bigger policy changes. Beyond that, understanding the fine details of trauma, adjusting to new cultures, and old beliefs allows for a truly full and patient-centered way of caring. By holding onto these ideas, mental health professionals can greatly improve how patients connect with care, make treatment results better, and help create a fairer and more welcoming health care system. The constant building of self-awareness, along with a promise to keep learning and speaking up for system changes, will give nurses and therapists the power to provide truly life-changing mental health care in a multicultural world.

References

1. Sue, D. W., & Sue, D. (2013). *Counseling the culturally diverse: Theory and practice* (6th ed.). John Wiley & Sons. [1]

2. Tervalon, M., & Murray-Garcia, J. (1998). Cultural humility versus cultural competence: A critical distinction in defining physician training outcomes in multicultural education. *Journal of Health Care for the Poor and Underserved*, 9(2), 117-125. [2]

3. American Psychological Association. (2017). *Guidelines for psychological practice with transgender and gender nonconforming people*. American Psychological Association. [3]

4. National Academies of Sciences, Engineering, and Medicine. (2017). *Understanding and addressing the root causes of health disparities: Proceedings of a workshop*. The National Academies Press. [4]

5. Cross, T. L., Bazron, B. J., Dennis, K. W., & Isaacs, M. R. (1989). *Toward a culturally competent system of care, Volume I: A monograph on effective services for minority children who are severely emotionally disturbed*. Georgetown University Child Development Center, CASSP Technical Assistance Center. [5]

6. Pew Research Center. (2019). *Religion & Public Life*. [6]

7. Bhugra, D., & Bhui, K. (2007). *Textbook of cultural psychiatry*. Cambridge University Press. [7]

8. Kleinman, A., Eisenberg, L., & Good, B. (1978). Culture, illness, and care: Clinical lessons from anthropologic and cross-cultural research. *Annals of Internal Medicine*, 88(2), 251-258. [8]

9. Raval, H., & Smith, M. (2003). Cultural competence: An essential requirement in culturally diverse societies. *Journal of Psychiatric and Mental Health Nursing*, 10(6), 660-667. [9]

10. Lu, F. G., Lim, R. F., & Mezzich, J. E. (1995). Issues in the assessment and diagnosis of Asian Americans: A cultural formulation approach. *Psychiatric Clinics of North America*, 18(3), 629-652. [10]

11. World Health Organization. (2008). *The global burden of disease: 2004 update*. WHO Press. [11]

12. Kirmayer, L. J., & Minas, H. (2000). The future of cultural psychiatry: An international perspective. *Canadian Journal of Psychiatry*, 45(5), 438-446. [12]

13. Sue, S., Zane, N., & Young, K. (1994). Research on psychotherapy with culturally diverse populations: A review and conclusions. In A. E. Bergin & S. L. Garfield (Eds.), *Handbook of psychotherapy and behavior change* (4th ed., pp. 783-817). John Wiley & Sons. [13]

14. Metzl, J. M. (2009). *The protest psychosis: How schizophrenia became a Black disease*. Beacon Press. [14]

15. Lewis-Fernández, R., & Díaz, N. (2003). The cultural formulation approach to psychiatric diagnosis: An update of the DSM-IV outline for cultural formulation. *Psychiatric Clinics of North America*, 26(3), 579-601. [15]

16. Flores, G., Abreu, M., Barone, C. P., Masur, E. K., & Horowitz, M. (2002). Errors of medical interpretation and their medical consequences in pediatric encounters. *Pediatrics*, 110(5), e67-e67. [16]

17. The Joint Commission. (2010). *Improving patient safety: Joint Commission issues new requirements to improve safety and quality of care for patients with limited English proficiency.* [17]

18. Griner, D., & Smith, T. B. (2006). Culturally adapted mental health intervention: A meta-analytic review. *Counselling Psychology Quarterly*, 19(4), 405-432. [18]

19. Benish, S. G., Quintana, S. M., & Wampold, B. E. (2011). Culturally adapted psychotherapy is more effective than nonadapted psychotherapy: A meta-analysis of studies. *Journal of Counseling Psychology*, 58(3), 282-294. [19]

20. Tran, N., Ta, V. P., & Ta, N. T. (2013). Family influence on mental health help-seeking attitudes among Vietnamese Americans. *Journal of Multicultural Counseling and Development*, 41(4), 226-237. [20]

21. Kirchheiner, J., & Brockmöller, J. (2005). Clinical consequences of cytochrome P450 2D6 genotypes on drug metabolism. *Clinical Pharmacology & Therapeutics*, 77(1), 1-12. [21]

22. U.S. Food and Drug Administration. (2020). *Table of Pharmacogenomic Biomarkers in Drug Labeling*. [22]

23. Turrini, G., Purgato, M., Ballette, F., Nosè, M., Ostuzzi, G., & Barbui, C. (2017). Asylum seekers and refugees: A systematic review of prevalence of and risk factors for mental disorders. *PLoS One*, 12(5), e0177701. [23]

24. Fazel, M., Reed, R. V., Panter-Brick, D., & Stein, A. (2018). Mental health of refugees. *The Lancet Psychiatry*, 5(6), 441-443. [24]

25. Asylum Protection Centre. (2023). *Asylum Seekers Living in Poverty*. [25]

26. Truth and Reconciliation Commission of Canada. (2015). *Honouring the Truth, Reconciling for the Future: Summary of the Final Report of the Truth and Reconciliation Commission of Canada*. [26]

27. Waldram, J. B., Herring, D. A., & Young, T. K. (2006). *Aboriginal health in Canada: Historical, cultural, and epidemiological perspectives* (2nd ed.). University of Toronto Press. [27]

28. Brave Heart, M. Y. H., & DeBruyn, L. M. (1998). The American Indian Holocaust: Healing historical trauma and cultural grief. *AIAN Journal of Health*, 7(1), 56-78. [28]

29. The Trevor Project. (2023). *2023 National Survey on LGBTQ Youth Mental Health*. [29]

30. Centers for Disease Control and Prevention. (2023). *Disability and Health Promotion*. [30]

31. FitzGerald, C., & Hurst, S. (2017). Implicit bias in healthcare professionals: A systematic review. *BMC Medical Ethics*, 18(1), 19. [31]

32. Hoffman, K. M., Trawalter, S., Axt, A. R., & Oliver, M. N. (2016). Racial bias in pain assessment and treatment recommendations, and false beliefs about biological differences between Blacks and Whites. *Proceedings of the National Academy of Sciences*, 113(16), 4296-4301. [32]

33. Mental Health America. (2023). *The State of Mental Health in America*. [33]

34. National Alliance on Mental Illness (NAMI). (2023). *Mental Health by the Numbers: Asian American and Pacific Islander*. [34]

35. American Psychological Association. (2022). *Demographics of the U.S. Psychology Workforce*. [35]

36. National Association of Social Workers. (2017). *Code of Ethics*. [36]

37. American Counseling Association. (2014). *ACA Code of Ethics*. [37]

38. American Nurses Association. (2015). *Code of Ethics for Nurses with Interpretive Statements*. [38]

39. Figley, C. R. (1995). *Compassion fatigue: Coping with secondary traumatic stress disorder in those who treat the traumatized*. Brunner/Mazel. [39]

40. Saakvitne, K. W., & Pearlman, L. A. (1996). *Transforming the pain: A workbook for vicarious traumatization*. W. W. Norton & Company. [40]

41. Maslach, C., & Leiter, M. P. (2016). *The truth about burnout: How organizations cause personal stress and what to do about it*. Jossey-Bass. [41]

42. Rössler, W., & Jaeger, M. (2006). The value of clinical supervision in psychotherapy. *Current Opinion in Psychiatry*, 19(5), 522-527. [42]

43. Sue, D. W. (2017). *The culturally competent counselor*. John Wiley & Sons. [43]

www.ingramcontent.com/pod-product-compliance
Lightning Source LLC
Chambersburg PA
CBHW070905280326
41934CB00008B/1594